Esophageal Function Testing

Editor

JOHN E. PANDOLFINO

GASTROINTESTINAL ENDOSCOPY CLINICS OF NORTH AMERICA

www.giendo.theclinics.com

Consulting Editor
CHARLES J. LIGHTDALE

October 2014 • Volume 24 • Number 4

ELSEVIER

1600 John F. Kennedy Boulevard • Suite 1800 • Philadelphia, Pennsylvania, 19103-2899

http://www.theclinics.com

GASTROINTESTINAL ENDOSCOPY CLINICS OF NORTH AMERICA Volume 24, Number 4
October 2014 ISSN 1052-5157, ISBN-13: 978-0-323-32609-4

Editor: Kerry Holland
Developmental Editor: Donald Mumford

Gastrointestinal Endoscopy Clinics of North America (ISSN 1052-5157) is published quarterly by Elsevier Inc., 360 Park Avenue South, New York, NY 10010-1710. Months of issue are January, April, July, and October. Business and Editorial Offices: 1600 John F. Kennedy Blvd., Suite 1800, Philadelphia, PA, 19103-2899. Periodicals postage paid at New York, NY and additional mailing offices. Subscription prices are $335.00 per year for US individuals, $486.00 per year for US institutions, $175.00 per year for US students and residents, $370.00 per year for Canadian individuals, $576.00 per year for Canadian institutions, $465.00 per year for international individuals, $576.00 per year for international institutions, and $245.00 per year for Canadian and foreign students/residents. To receive student/resident rate, orders must be accompanied by name of affiliated institution, date of term, and the *signature* of program/residency coordinator on institution letterhead. Orders will be billed at individual rate until proof of status is received. Foreign air speed delivery is included in all *Clinics* subscription prices. All prices are subject to change without notice. **POSTMASTER:** Send address change to *Gastrointestinal Endoscopy Clinics of North America*, Elsevier Health Sciences Division, Subscription Customer Service, 3251 Riverport Lane, Maryland Heights, MO 63043. **Customer Service: 1-800-654-2452 (US). From outside the United States, call 1-314-447-8871. Fax: 1-314-447-8029. E-mail: JournalsCustomerService-usa@elsevier.com (for print support) or JournalsOnlineSupport-usa@elsevier.com (for online support).**

Reprints. For copies of 100 or more, of articles in this publication, please contact the Commercial Reprints Department, Elsevier Inc., 360 Park Avenue South, New York, NY 10010-1710. Tel. 212-633-3874; Fax: 212-633-3820; E-mail: reprints@elsevier.com.

Gastrointestinal Endoscopy Clinics of North America is covered in *Excerpta Medica, MEDLINE/PubMed (Index Medicus), and MEDLINE/MEDLARS.*

Contributors

CONSULTING EDITOR

CHARLES J. LIGHTDALE, MD
Professor of Medicine, Division of Digestive and Liver Diseases, Columbia University Medical Center, New York, New York

EDITOR

JOHN E. PANDOLFINO, MD, MSci
Professor, Department of Medicine, Division of Gastroenterology and Hepatology, Feinberg School of Medicine, Northwestern University, Chicago, Illinois

AUTHORS

GUY BOECKXSTAENS, MD, PhD
Department of Gastroenterology, Translational Research Center for Gastrointestinal Disorders (TARGID), University Hospital of Leuven, Catholic University of Leuven, Leuven, Belgium

ALBERT J. BREDENOORD, MD
Department of Gastroenterology and Hepatology, Academic Medical Center Amsterdam, Amsterdam, The Netherlands

C. PRAKASH GYAWALI, MD, MRCP
Professor of Medicine, Division of Gastroenterology, Washington University School of Medicine, Saint Louis, Missouri

MICHELLE S. HAN, MD
Research Fellow, Department of Surgery, University of Rochester Medical Center, University of Rochester, Rochester, New York

PETER J. KAHRILAS, MD, AGAF
Professor, Department of Medicine, Feinberg School of Medicine, Northwestern University, Chicago, Illinois

DAVID A. KATZKA, MD
Professor of Medicine, Division of Gastroenterology and Hepatology, Mayo Clinic, Rochester, Minnesota

PHILIP B. MINER Jr, MD
Clinical Professor of Medicine, Division of Gastroenterology, Department of Medicine; President and Medical Director, Oklahoma Foundation for Digestive Research, Oklahoma University School of Medicine, Oklahoma City, Oklahoma

RAVINDER K. MITTAL, MD
Professor of Medicine, Division of Gastroenterology, Department of Medicine, San Diego VA Health Care System, and University of California, San Diego, California

AN MOONEN, MD
Department of Gastroenterology, Translational Research Center for Gastrointestinal
Disorders (TARGID), University Hospital of Leuven, Catholic University of Leuven, Leuven,
Belgium

SALMAN NUSRAT, MD
Fellow in Gastroenterology, Section of Digestive Disease and Nutrition, Department of
Medicine, University of Oklahoma Health Sciences Center, Oklahoma City, Oklahoma

JOHN E. PANDOLFINO, MD, MSci
Professor, Department of Medicine, Division of Gastroenterology and Hepatology,
Feinberg School of Medicine, Northwestern University, Chicago, Illinois

AMIT PATEL, MD
Division of Gastroenterology, Washington University School of Medicine, Saint Louis,
Missouri

JEFFREY H. PETERS, MD, FACS
Chief Operating Officer, Department of Surgery, University Hospitals, Cleveland, Ohio

SABINE ROMAN, MD, PhD
Associate Professor, Digestive Physiology, Hôpital E Herriot, Hospices Civils de Lyon,
Claude Bernard Lyon I University, Lyon, France

CAROLINE M.G. SALEH, MS
Department of Gastroenterology and Hepatology, Academic Medical Center Amsterdam,
Amsterdam, The Netherlands

DANIEL SIFRIM, MD, PhD
Centre for Digestive Diseases, Barts and the London School of Medicine and Dentistry,
Queen Mary University of London; Gastrointestinal Physiology Unit, Barts Health NHS
Trust, Royal London Hospital, London, United Kingdom

RADU TUTUIAN, MD, PhD
Division of Gastroenterology, University Clinics of Visceral Surgery and Medicine, Bern
University Hospital – Inselspital Bern, Bern, Switzerland; Division of Gastroenterology,
Spital Region Oberaargau (SRO) – Langenthal, Langenthal, Switzerland

MARCELO F. VELA, MD, MSCR
Associate Professor of Medicine, Division of Gastroenterology, Mayo Clinic Arizona,
Scottsdale, Arizona

PHILIP WOODLAND, MBBS, PhD
Centre for Digestive Diseases, Barts and the London School of Medicine and Dentistry,
Queen Mary University of London; Gastrointestinal Physiology Unit, Barts Health NHS
Trust, Royal London Hospital, London, United Kingdom

YINGLIAN XIAO, MD, PhD
Associate Professor, Department of Gastroenterology and Hepatology, The First Affiliated
Hospital, Sun Yat-sen University, Guangzhou, China

ETSURO YAZAKI, PhD, MAGIP
Centre for Digestive Diseases, Barts and the London School of Medicine and Dentistry,
Queen Mary University of London; Gastrointestinal Physiology Unit, Barts Health NHS
Trust, Royal London Hospital, London, United Kingdom

Contents

High-resolution manometry (HRM) has advanced the understanding of esophageal peristaltic mechanisms and has simplified esophageal motor testing. In this article the technical aspects of HRM are addressed, focusing on test protocols, in addition to concerns and pitfalls in performing esophageal motor studies. Specifically, catheter positioning, equipment-related artifacts, basal data acquisition, adequate swallows, and provocative maneuvers are discussed.

The Chicago Classification defines esophageal motility disorders in high resolution manometry. This is based on individual scoring of 10 swallows performed in supine position. Disorders of esophago-gastric junction (EGJ) outflow obstruction are defined by a median integrated relaxation pressure above the limit of normal and divided into 3 achalasia subtypes and EGJ outflow obstruction. Major motility disorders (aperistalsis, distal esophageal spasm, and hypercontractile esophagus) are patterns not encountered in controls in the context of normal EGJ relaxation. Finally with the latest version of the Chicago Classification, only two minor motor disorders are considered: ineffective esophageal motility and fragmented peristalsis.

Barium esophagography, although an old test, remains important to the understanding of esophageal physiology and diagnosis of esophageal disorders. It provides additive and/or confirmatory information to endoscopy and is the more accurate means of yielding diagnosis. Barium esophagography allows correlation of symptoms with barium findings and with varied textures substances. It allows, particularly for oropharyngeal dysfunction, implementation therapeutic maneuvers and instructions while testing. The caveat to maintaining the benefits of barium esophagography is continuing to promote and support expertise from our radiologists in performing these studies, which has been challenged by our cost-efficient and high-tech medical society.

The development and advancement of ambulatory esophageal pH monitoring has provided a key tool with which pathologic esophageal acid exposure can be objectively measured; although not perfect, it provides the clinician with arguably the most important piece of information in the diagnosis and management of patients with gastroesophageal reflux disease. It is also important to emphasize that, although esophageal pH monitoring can reliably measure esophageal acid exposure, assessing the relationship of abnormal findings and the patients' symptoms is a much more complex matter and, of course, the key to successful treatment outcomes.

The function of the esophagus is transporting nutrients from the oropharyngeal cavity to the stomach. This is achieved by coordinated contractions and relaxation of the tubular esophagus and the upper and lower esophageal sphincter. Multichannel intraluminal impedance monitoring offers quantification of esophageal bolus transit and/or retention without the use of ionizing radiation. Combined with conventional or high-resolution manometry, impedance measurements complement the quantification of esophageal body contraction and sphincter relaxation, offering a more comprehensive evaluation of esophageal function. Further studies evaluating the utility of quantifying bolus transit will help clarify the role and position of impedance measurements.

The mechanical properties of the esophagogastric junction (EGJ) are of major importance for the competence of the EGJ. Although manometry reliably measures sphincter pressure, no information is provided on distensibility, a crucial determinant of flow across the EGJ. Recently, a new technique, impedance planimetry, was introduced allowing accurate measurement of compliance or distensibility. This review discusses the recent advances in this area and highlights the clinical relevance of this new technique evaluating the mechanical properties of the esophageal wall and EGJ.

Dramatic progress has been made over the past decade in the sophistication and availability of equipment to test esophageal motility and sensation. High-resolution esophageal manometry and impedance have moved from the research clinic into clinical practice. Some of the testing is costly and time consuming, and requires extensive experience to perform the testing and properly interpret the results. These sensory studies are valuable in the interpretation of clinical problems, and provide important research information. Clinicians should evaluate the research studies to advance their understanding of the pathophysiology of the esophagus.

Rumination is a phenomenon characterized by retrograde flow of gastric contents into the mouth, otherwise known as regurgitation. Repetitive excessive occurrence of rumination is considered pathologic and is known as the rumination syndrome. Belching occurs occasionally in everyone and is often not related to a disease or a pathologic condition. Gastric belches are physiologic events caused by retrograde flow of air into the esophagus and mouth; however, supragastric belching is associated with belching disorders and is considered pathologic behavior.

Esophageal function testing should be used for differential diagnosis of dysphagia. Dysphagia can be the consequence of hypermotility or hypomotility of the muscles of the esophagus. Decreased esophageal or esophagogastric junction distensibility can provoke dysphagia. The most well established esophageal dysmotility is achalasia. Other motility disorders can also cause dysphagia. High-resolution manometry (HRM) is the gold standard investigation for esophageal motility disorders. Simultaneous measurement of HRM and intraluminal impedance can be useful to assess motility and bolus transit. Impedance planimetry measures distensibility of the esophageal body and gastroesophageal junction in patients with achalasia and eosinophilic esophagitis.

Gastroesophageal reflux disease (GERD) is frequently diagnosed by symptoms and good response to acid suppression with proton pump inhibitors. Further work up is required when the diagnosis of GERD is uncertain, for alarm symptoms, PPI-refractoriness, and often for extraesophageal presentations. Useful tools include endoscopy for mucosal assessment and reflux monitoring (pH or impedance-pH) to quantify reflux burden. Objective documentation of pathological reflux is mandatory prior to anti-reflux surgery. In some patients, symptoms that can be attributed to GERD may have other causes; in these patients, testing that excludes GERD helps direct the diagnostic and treatment efforts to other causes.

Manometry and impedance provide only surrogate information regarding longitudinal wall function and are focused on contractile amplitude and lumen content. Ultrasound imaging provides a unique perspective of esophageal function by providing important information regarding longitudinal muscle contraction. Laser Doppler assessment of perfusion may be an important complementary tool to assess abnormal wall blood perfusion as a possible mechanism of pain.

GASTROINTESTINAL ENDOSCOPY CLINICS OF NORTH AMERICA

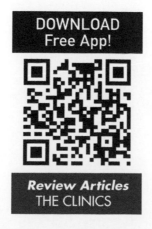

DOWNLOAD Free App!

Review Articles
THE CLINICS

NOW AVAILABLE FOR YOUR iPhone and iPad

Foreword

New and Improved Methods for Esophageal Function Testing

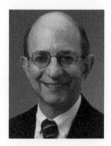

Charles J. Lightdale, MD
Consulting Editor

Dysphagia, refractory heartburn, reflux, chest pain, and dyspepsia are among the most common upper gastrointestinal complaints that elicit referral to gastroenterologists. Upper gastrointestinal endoscopy is usually the first-line test to identify diseases that can be diagnosed by visualization and pathologic studies of endoscopic biopsies. In some cases, however, endoscopy is not diagnostic. Fortunately, in recent years there have been tremendous advances in esophageal function testing, which can provide specific diagnoses to explain symptoms pointing to an esophageal origin. It is obviously very important for gastroenterologists to understand and properly utilize these new and improved tests, increasingly performed by specialists with a focused interest in esophageal diseases.

The editor for this issue of the *Gastrointestinal Endoscopy Clinics of North America* devoted to esophageal function testing is Dr John Pandolfino, Chief, Division of Medicine-Gastroenterology and Hepatology at Northwestern University Feinberg School of Medicine. Dr Pandolfino has been in the forefront of the field of esophageal and swallowing disorders and has gathered an extraordinary array of experts who provide a remarkably clear state-of-the-art compilation, with a look into the near future as well. This issue represents a terrific resource not only for specialists in the field ("esophagologists") but also for clinical gastroenterologists in general and should not be missed.

Charles J. Lightdale, MD
Division of Digestive and Liver Diseases
Columbia University Medical Center
161 Fort Washington Avenue
New York, NY 10032, USA

E-mail address:
CJL18@columbia.edu

Gastrointest Endoscopy Clin N Am 24 (2014) xi
http://dx.doi.org/10.1016/j.giec.2014.07.004
1052-5157/14/$ – see front matter © 2014 Elsevier Inc. All rights reserved.

Preface
Esophageal Function Testing

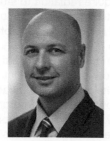

John E. Pandolfino, MD, MSci
Editor

It is my pleasure to serve as the guest editor for a special issue of *Gastrointestinal Endoscopy Clinics of North America* that is devoted to the topic of esophageal function testing. Although at first glance it would seem that this topic would not fit with the typical subject matter of this particular publication, it is important to realize that esophageal function tests are complementary to endoscopy in exploring esophageal complaints. In fact, a prerequisite for performing many of these studies is a negative endoscopy, and thus the endoscopist should be well-informed regarding the indication and utility of these tests. In addition, some of these newer technologies now require endoscopy to be performed during the study as the placement or positioning of the measurement tool will require endoscopic landmarks or direct visualization during placement.

In addition, a review on esophageal function testing is also timely as there have been major advances in most of the older techniques, and new novel methodologies have been developed that allow for a more visual and accurate description of physiologic and anatomical data. My goals for this issue are to provide a comprehensive review of all of the available technologies and to focus the discussion on how these techniques can impact clinical practice and research into the pathogenesis of esophageal diseases. In addition, I've also asked my collaborators of this issue to provide background on the technical aspects of these devices as this is extremely important in determining which test is most appropriate for a specific complaint.

With this in mind, the issue begins with a description of the technical aspects of manometry as this is the quintessential esophageal function test, and there have been dramatic improvements in this technology over the last decade. The introduction of high-resolution manometry by Ray Clouse and his team at Washington University, St. Louis, has revolutionized our evaluation of esophageal motor disorders. This is highlighted in the second article, which provides an update on a new classification scheme, "The Chicago Classification," that utilizes esophageal pressure topography to display and analyze esophageal motor function. Although the next article appears

1052-5157/14/$ – see front matter © 2014 Published by Elsevier Inc.
giendo.theclinics.com

to be a step backwards as it focuses on an older technique, one must recognize that the barium esophagram is still an important tool in the assessment of esophageal diseases, and it sometimes can be an important arbiter of equivocal cases.

The next two articles focus on techniques to study gastroesophageal reflux. Impedance monitoring provides an alternative to techniques that require radiation to study bolus transit and thus is a useful tool for ambulatory reflux testing. This technique has become important in the assessment of patients not responding to proton pump inhibitor therapy. However, pH testing still remains an important component in the evaluation of gastroesophageal reflux disease and the accompanying article focuses on the value of this surrogate marker for reflux and how adapting this into a wireless modality and combined impedance–pH system could help improve accuracy. Complementing these two articles is an important review of postprandial symptoms that may mimic refractory reflux, and this article highlights how rumination and supragastric belching can be differentiated from gastroesophageal reflux disease using novel techniques that combine manometry and impedance.

This issue also emphasizes new technologies that are less mainstream and are more prominently used in research. The functional lumen imaging probe represents a high-resolution impedance planimetry system that can provide information regarding the mechanical properties of the esophageal wall and the esophagogastric junction. In addition, new testing modalities and imaging techniques such as sensitivity testing and functional MRI are providing exciting information regarding the role of visceral hypersensitivity and central processing of esophageal stimuli in symptom generation. The role of these techniques is emerging and it is likely that this work will give rise to a new generation of esophageal function tests.

Anchoring the issue are three final articles that seek to provide a cohesive approach to patients presenting with dysphagia and reflux and a glimpse into the future beyond manometry and impedance. Dysphagia is a complaint that typically begins with endoscopy to rule out mechanical causes for dysphagia, and a systematic approach is provided to help guide decisions focused on managing these patients. Similarly, the management of GERD is also approached in the context of a negative endoscopy as reflux testing and manometry should be performed after a negative examination to look for an alternative diagnosis or documentation that the patient is truly refractory to medical management. Each of these reviews also highlights the limitations of our current strategies, and this is a nice segue into the final article that looks at novel techniques that could potentially complement our current strategies in the future.

I hope that you will find the information in this issue both informative and useful in terms of improving the management of patients with a negative endoscopy or equivocal findings. This issue of *Gastrointestinal Endoscopy Clinics of North America* would not have been possible without the excellent contributions of my friends and colleagues, and I am eternally grateful for their effort and time.

John E. Pandolfino, MD, MSci
Department of Medicine
Division of Gastroenterology and Hepatology
Feinberg School of Medicine
Northwestern University
676 St Clair Street, 14th Floor
Chicago, IL 60611-2951, USA

E-mail address:
j-pandolfino@northwestern.edu

Esophageal Motor Function
Technical Aspects of Manometry

C. Prakash Gyawali, MD, MRCP*, Amit Patel, MD

KEYWORDS

- High-resolution manometry • Clouse plot • Esophageal motor function • Dysphagia

KEY POINTS

- High-resolution manometry (HRM) affords easier identification of anatomic landmarks and esophageal motor patterns, shorter duration of procedures, uniform analysis parameters, and better comprehension for learners in comparison with conventional manometry.
- HRM is used to evaluate esophageal motor function in patients with esophageal symptoms unexplained after endoscopy or contrast studies, to assess esophageal peristalsis before foregut surgery, and to localize the lower esophageal sphincter (LES) for placement of pH and pH-impedance catheters.
- Aberrancies in catheter positioning, such as failure to traverse the LES or the diaphragm, and equipment-related artifacts, such as thermal drift or sensor malfunction, should be recognized and rectified appropriately.
- The technician performing the HRM study needs to be able to reassure the patient, identify esophageal landmarks and motor patterns, understand critical and noncritical imperfections, and modify the study accordingly.

INTRODUCTION

Esophageal manometry consists of measurement of pressure events in the esophagus following test swallows, represented as timing and amplitude of pressure events.[1] Esophageal intraluminal pressures are converted to an electrical signal that can be recorded, amplified, and displayed as pressure tracings at each recording location along the esophagus. Initial conventional manometry systems consisted of an array of unidirectional recording sites distributed at predefined locations along the length of a catheter placed in the esophageal lumen. Line tracings of pressure events were displayed in a stacked format from proximal to distal esophagus, and proximal stomach. The characteristics of the pressure events designated whether

Division of Gastroenterology, Washington University School of Medicine, 660 South Euclid Avenue, Campus Box 8124, Saint Louis, MO 63110, USA
* Corresponding author.
E-mail address: cprakash@dom.wustl.edu

Gastrointest Endoscopy Clin N Am 24 (2014) 527–543
http://dx.doi.org/10.1016/j.giec.2014.06.003   giendo.theclinics.com

the esophageal body, an esophageal sphincter, or the gastric baseline was addressed by each recording site.[1]

High-resolution manometry (HRM) represents a paradigm shift from conventional manometry in that multiple circumferential pressure sensors are used and topographic plots of esophageal pressure data are generated. These plots can be viewed as colored contour maps on which each color represents a pressure value. The close spacing of sensors allows better sampling of esophageal intraluminal pressures as a continuum throughout the esophagus and its sphincters, rather than as point samples at predefined distances as used with conventional manometry.[2,3] Computerized software programs fill points in between pressure recordings with best-fit data to create smooth color-contour plots of esophageal peristalsis, now uniformly termed Clouse plots in honor of Ray Clouse who pioneered the technology (**Fig. 1**).[2,4] Advantages of HRM over conventional manometry include easier identification of anatomic landmarks, shorter duration of data acquisition, more specific assessment of sphincter function, and easier recognition of motor patterns.[1]

INDICATIONS AND CONTRAINDICATIONS

HRM represents the test of choice to evaluate esophageal motor function. The primary value of HRM remains the identification of esophageal outflow obstruction from a motor process such as achalasia. The benefit stems primarily from the fact that software tools have been designed to extract nadir pressures during expected lower esophageal sphincter (LES) relaxation during a test swallow. Of these, the integrated relaxation pressure (IRP), which extracts 4 seconds of continuous or discontinuous nadir pressure, performs the best.[5] The sensitivity of IRP as an HRM tool for the diagnosis of achalasia has been well documented in comparisons with point-pressure sensors

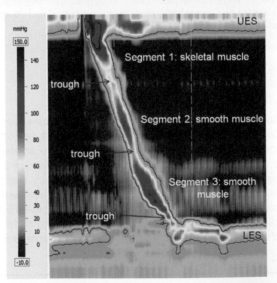

Fig. 1. Clouse plot showing a normal peristaltic sequence following a test swallow. The x-axis represents time, the y-axis represents length along the esophagus, and contraction amplitudes are depicted as color contours, with warmer colors representing higher amplitudes. High-resolution manometry has demonstrated esophageal peristalsis to consist of a chain of relaxing sphincters (LES, lower esophageal sphincter; UES, upper esophageal sphincter) and contracting segments (segment 1: skeletal muscle; segments 2 and 3: smooth muscle), separated by pressure troughs.

and sleeve sensors.[5] In addition, motor mechanisms involved in postfundoplication dysphagia can be evaluated using HRM.

HRM is frequently performed for assessment of esophageal symptoms not fully explained by endoscopic or radiologic studies (**Box 1**). Both hypermotility disorders (spastic processes such as distal esophageal spasm or jackhammer esophagus) and hypomotility disorders (aperistalsis, frequent failed peristalsis) may be identified in these settings. HRM assessment of the upper esophageal sphincter (UES) may complement other modalities of assessment of pharyngeal and proximal esophageal peristalsis and function. The most frequent use of esophageal manometry is in localization of the proximal border of the LES for placement of pH and pH-impedance probes.

High-grade oropharyngeal or esophageal obstruction from a structural process could preclude placement of the motility catheter, and constitute an absolute contraindication to esophageal motor testing. Patients on chronic anticoagulation are generally asked to hold their anticoagulants for 3 to 5 days because of the risk for epistaxis. The indication for the procedure should be carefully assessed in patients with profound disorders of coagulation and those with significant risk of aspiration (although dry swallows could be obtained in the latter setting). Other indications and contraindications for esophageal manometry are summarized in **Box 1**.

Box 1
Indications and contraindications for esophageal motility testing

Indications

Transit symptoms (dysphagia, regurgitation) with no structural process identified on endoscopy and/or barium contrast studies

Abnormal esophageal emptying identified on endoscopy and/or barium contrast studies

Esophageal symptoms (chest pain, regurgitation, heartburn) with no structural explanation and no benefit from empiric acid suppression

Transit symptoms following foregut surgery, especially fundoplication

Transit symptoms following bariatric procedures, especially laparoscopic band placement

Localization of the lower esophageal sphincter for placement of pH and pH-impedance probes

Assessment of esophageal peristaltic function before fundoplication

Dysphagia localized to the proximal esophagus and upper esophageal sphincter

Contraindications

Absolute

    Esophageal obstruction from an infiltrating process such as a tumor

    Abnormal nasal passages preventing catheter insertion

    Abnormal oropharyngeal anatomy

    Frank aspiration with water swallows (dry swallows can be obtained)

    Significantly abnormal coagulation parameters

Relative

    Patients on chronic anticoagulation (anticoagulants can be held for 3–5 days)

    Inability to swallow on command (dry swallows can be obtained)

    Inability to tolerate the catheter (catheter can be sometimes placed at endoscopy, while sedated, if procedure is absolutely necessary)

THE PROCEDURE
Equipment Preparation

HRM catheters are made by several manufacturers, and can be either solid-state or water-perfused. Manufacturer instructions need to be followed for catheter calibration before initiation of the study. Water-perfused catheters need to be flushed with degassed water, and pressure measurements calibrated to the zero position, which is, the level of the esophagus with the patient lying on the stretcher.[6] With solid-state catheters, pressure calibration is performed before each study by applying known pressure to pressure sensors to ensure pressure readings are accurate; this is typically an automated process using a pressurized chamber into which the catheter is inserted.[1] Because solid-state sensors can be affected by temperature, intermittent calibration using a water bath at 37°C is recommended, so that a pressure correction can be calculated for pressures recorded at body temperature when calibration is performed at room temperature. This thermal compensation is applied at the end of the procedure.[7]

Supplies needed for esophageal manometry include syringes with distilled or tap water for test swallows, a cup with a drinking straw containing water, a kidney tray and towels in case the patient retches or vomits, cotton-tipped swabs, KY jelly for catheter lubrication, lidocaine jelly for topical anesthesia of the nasal passages, and tape for securing the catheter after intubation. If viscous or solid boluses are to be administered, appropriate food items (eg, viscous jelly, yogurt, bread, marshmallows) need to be at hand.

Some manufacturers of HRM catheters recommend using a protective sheath over the solid-state catheter to simplify disinfection protocols between procedures; these cannot be used with catheters containing impedance sensors.[1]

Patient Preparation

Esophageal manometry is best performed in a well-lit room with a comfortable ambience. The patient changes into a gown that covers the chest and torso. Preprocedure symptom questionnaires and requisition forms are completed as the catheter and equipment are readied. The HRM operator first explains the procedure to the patient, and describes why the procedure is being performed. The operator reassures and engages the patient, describes what the patient can expect, and uses distractive measures in case there is oropharyngeal discomfort or gagging.[8] Knowledge of anatomic abnormalities, such as hiatal hernia, suspicion of a dilated esophagus, and prior foregut surgery, may assist in preparing for and performing the procedure.[9]

Patients should have nothing to eat or drink for at least 6 hours (clear liquids for 2–3 days may be needed if achalasia is suspected) before the HRM study to prevent aspiration of gastric or esophageal contents. Medications that affect esophageal motility (caffeine-containing medications, prokinetics, nitrates, calcium-channel blockers, anticholinergics, opiates, and tricyclic antidepressants) are best avoided whenever possible, and should be decided on a case-by-case basis in the context of the clinical indication for the study and potential impact on patient management. Allergies to analgesics must be documented, as topical anesthesia with lidocaine spray and/or viscous lidocaine is used in the nasal passages in many centers to minimize discomfort and maximize the success of nasal intubation.[1]

Patient Positioning

The esophageal motility catheter is best inserted with patients sitting upright and facing the operator. The head is tilted up slightly to allow the operator to visualize the nasal passages before insertion. After adequate positioning of the catheter, the patient is asked to lie down in a supine position, as esophageal peristalsis is traditionally assessed without the effect of gravity on bolus transit. Furthermore, with conventional manometry using pneumohydraulic pumps, pressure needed to be zeroed to the position of the catheter, which required a horizontal position. The head end of the bed is typically tilted upward by 10° to 15°, and the patient is asked to lean slightly to the left to assist with swallowing of water boluses that are squirted into the mouth.[1,10]

Upright patient positioning is now possible using HRM, as zeroing of pressure to patient position is not necessary. The upright, seated position may be better tolerated by patients with severe esophageal dysmotility, thereby minimizing the risk of regurgitation and aspiration in comparison with the supine position. Normative upright pressure values exist, and have been compared with the supine position.[11] Peristalsis is more coordinated and vigorous, with a slower contraction front velocity in the supine position.[11] Motor diagnoses are reported to be generally concordant in more than 70% of cases between supine and upright positions; discordant cases were mostly accounted for by an excess of hypomotility disorders in the upright position.[12] However, numeric reduction in IRP and contraction vigor is seen in the sitting position, with others reporting reclassification of esophageal outflow obstruction in approximately 10%, leading some investigators to suggest performing up to 5 swallows in the upright position in most patients.

Catheter Insertion

A cup containing water, with a straw for sipping, is provided to the patient, as swallowing of water during catheter advancement reduces patient discomfort. The catheter tip is lubricated and passed through the nasal passages with the chin tilted slightly upward. When the patient feels the catheter at the back of the throat, the neck can be flexed and the catheter inserted into the esophagus while the patient takes small sips of water to maintain relaxation of the UES and, subsequently, the LES.[1] Having patients open their mouths, watch the Clouse plots on the screen, or squeeze a soft ball can help focus attention away from discomfort or gagging.[9]

Catheter Positioning

When properly positioned, the HRM catheter extends from the pharynx to the stomach, with at least 1 sensor in the pharynx and 3 sensors in the stomach. In the normal setting, the UES and LES/esophagogastric junction (EGJ) are visible as 2 bands of pressure (**Fig. 2**). The HRM operator is trained in identification of anatomic landmarks, including the UES, LES, and diaphragmatic crural impression. The diaphragmatic crural impression together with the LES constitutes the EGJ. The location of the diaphragmatic crura can be assessed by identifying pressure inversion with respiration; intrathoracic pressure is more negative during inspiration, whereas intra-abdominal pressure is more negative during expiration (see **Fig. 2**). If the diaphragmatic crural impression is not easily identified, the patient can be asked to take a deep breath, which will magnify these pressure changes. If the EGJ is not traversed by the HRM catheter, these pressure changes with breathing will not be seen; instead, a "butterfly" or mirror image may be seen, indicating that the catheter is curled up in the esophagus and requires repositioning (**Fig. 3**). Separation between the LES and diaphragmatic crura indicates the presence of a hiatus hernia.

If a pressurization pattern is seen that extends from the contraction front all the way to the bottom of the screen, air may be present in the catheter sheath if the Given HRM system is being used. The operator should remove the catheter and replace the sheath if the tracing looks unusual.

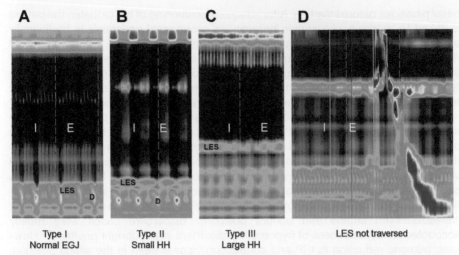

Fig. 2. Relationships between LES and esophagogastric junction (EGJ). (*A*) Normal EGJ (type I), with overlapping LES and diaphragmatic crura, and no separation between the two. (*B*) Type II hiatus hernia (HH) in which LES and diaphragmatic crura are not overlapping, but separation is less than 2 cm. (*C*) Type III: separation between LES and diaphragmatic crura; in this instance, the diaphragmatic crura have not been traversed. (*D*) LES is not traversed. When in doubt, this can be recognized when the patient is asked to swallow. D, diaphragm; E, esophagus.

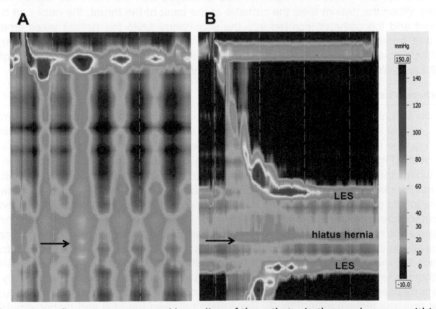

Fig. 3. Butterfly patterns generated by curling of the catheter in the esophagus or within a hiatus hernia. Arrows point to site where the catheter curls back up. (*A*) The catheter is curled up in the esophageal body in a patient with achalasia, with mirroring of esophageal body contraction above and below where the catheter curls. (*B*) The catheter traverses the LES and curls up within a hiatus hernia, with retrograde movement back up into the esophagus through the LES.

An inability to traverse the LES is a critical imperfection that needs to be recognized by the HRM operator in real time. Although this difficulty occurs most often in achalasia, the diagnosis of achalasia may still be made with similar frequency (up to 94%) as with perfect studies if the clinical context and other tests are reviewed.[13] Straightening and lengthening the esophagus by asking the patient to stand up, repositioning the catheter, or having the patient gulp water (which may allow the LES to relax) may help maneuver the catheter through the LES.[9] Regardless, several maneuvers can be used to attempt to traverse the LES (**Box 2**).

By contrast, not traversing the diaphragmatic crura is a noncritical imperfection. This difficulty typically occurs with large hiatal hernias. In this setting, if the LES is traversed there remains a small risk that LES metrics may be inaccurate if there is pressure compartmentalization within the hiatal hernia. However, esophageal body peristalsis and LES function can typically be ascertained adequately.[9] Insertion with the patient standing up may assist with traversing the diaphragm, as the hiatus hernia may reduce in this position. Alternatively, placing the HRM catheter under endoscopic guidance can be considered.

Once the resting pressures generated by the UES and LES are identified, the catheter is fixed in place by taping to the nose, and the patient is allowed to accommodate to the HRM catheter before initiating the study. This interval avoids artificial elevations of resting UES pressure and repeated dry swallowing.[10]

TECHNIQUE
Landmark Phase

Once the patient is comfortable with the manometry catheter in place, the standard manometry protocol begins with a baseline recording without swallow artifacts (typically 30 seconds in duration) to assess the resting characteristics of the UES and LES (landmark phase). Sometimes a patient swallows so frequently that the basal landmark phase cannot be optimally recorded (**Fig. 4**). In these instances of patients who are intolerant of the HRM catheter whereby a swallow-free and artifact-free landmark phase cannot be obtained within the first 5 minutes of the study, the landmark phase can be obtained at a convenient time later in the study, shortening the study duration without compromising quality.[14]

Adequate Swallows

A series of ten 5-mL room-temperature water swallows are administered in the supine position, at least 20 to 30 seconds apart.[1,6] This interval between swallows allows the resting LES pressure to return to baseline and avoids artifacts from swallow-induced suppression of esophageal motor activity (deglutitive inhibition).[15] The current interpretation algorithms are based on 10 water swallows, as dry swallows do not generate

---

Box 2

Placement of the motility catheter across the esophagogastric junction

- Catheter is advanced with patient standing up
- The patient raises arms above the head
- A 45° to 90° twist is applied counterclockwise on the catheter
- The patient takes repeated gulps of water
- The catheter is placed under endoscopic guidance

BEGINNING OF STUDY   END OF STUDY

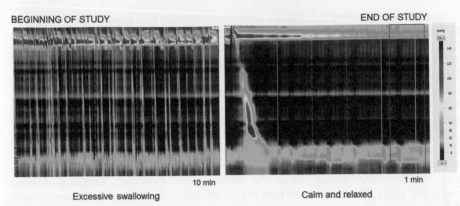

10 min   1 min

Excessive swallowing   Calm and relaxed

Fig. 4. Placement of the landmark phase. Although the landmark phase is typically placed at the beginning of the study, this may not be possible in anxious patients who may gag or not be able to refrain from swallowing to obtain the basal recording. In such instances, the patient may be more relaxed at the end of the study, when the landmark basal period can be recorded.

a swallow sequence similar to a wet swallow. Belching, gagging, double swallows, secondary peristaltic sequences, and transient LES relaxations also generate artifacts that the HRM operator needs to recognize; swallows in the vicinity of these artifacts should be rejected and new swallows obtained (**Fig. 5**).

The Chicago Classification algorithm for characterizing esophageal motor disorders is based on 10 water swallows in the supine position.[16] However, a lesser complement of adequate swallows can be tolerated, and interpretation is possible if at least 5 to 7 swallows are adequate. In a series of 2000 HRM studies, less than 7 evaluable swallows were seen in 12% of studies,[13] which did not compromise diagnoses of major motor disorders if the clinical context was applied. However, in another cohort of patients studied by this same group, as few as 5 swallows were adequate for reaching a diagnostic conclusion, except for diagnoses for which the number of swallows with abnormalities mattered.[17]

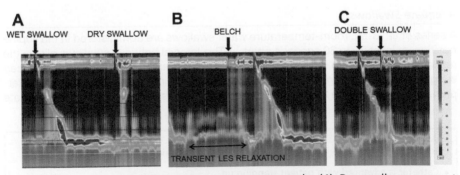

Fig. 5. Artifacts that may compromise a manometry study. (*A*) Dry swallows may not generate a normal peristaltic sequence even in normal healthy individuals, and should be rejected in favor of wet swallows 20 to 30 seconds apart. (*B*) Transient LES relaxations can occur during a manometry study, and need to be recognized by the operator so that test swallows are not performed within 20 to 30 seconds. Transient LES relaxations may be associated with belching or secondary peristaltic sequences. (*C*) Double swallows may generate disorganized peristaltic sequences, and should also be rejected.

Provocative Maneuvers

Provocative maneuvers are increasingly applied to clinical HRM. The simplest of these measures include multiple rapid swallows (MRS) (five 2-mL water swallows <3 seconds apart) and multiple water swallows (200 mL water within 30 seconds, also termed free water drinking).[18,19] Both of these maneuvers rely on intact deglutitive inhibition during the swallows, followed by an exaggerated contractile response following the last swallow of the sequence. Free water drinking also provides a volume load to the esophagus, which can result in esophageal pressurization if there is subtle outflow obstruction. MRS is most useful in assessing esophageal peristaltic reserve.[18] For instance, if contraction following MRS is suboptimal or absent, likelihood of late postoperative dysphagia is significantly higher than if adequate contraction is recorded.[18,19]

In achalasia spectrum disorders, when inhibitory dysfunction is profound and there is esophageal body aperistalsis, the LES does not relax during the inhibitory phase of MRS. By contrast, when esophageal body peristalsis is retained or spastic, partial LES relaxation can be identified.[20] In the presence of esophageal body pressurization and esophageal outflow obstruction, sphincter dysfunction and structural outflow obstruction can potentially be distinguished with provocative measures. In healthy individuals, both maneuvers result in profound and complete LES relaxation during the swallows from deglutitive inhibition. Although patients with achalasia lack these responses, those with structural outflow obstruction may demonstrate partial or complete LES relaxation, as deglutitive inhibition remains intact despite esophageal pressurization.[1]

Although the standard HRM protocol is performed with water swallows, this is not representative of real-world food ingestion. Viscous boluses such as applesauce or yogurt, solid boluses such as bread or marshmallows, and even test meals have been used during esophageal HRM with increased diagnostic yield of obstructive processes in limited circumstances. Increasing the consistency of the test bolus augments peristaltic vigor, although multiple swallows are more often needed to clear solid boluses from the esophagus, increasing the proportion of ineffective esophageal contractions.[21] Standardization of provocative measures may generate clinically useful diagnostic criteria in the future.

COMPLICATIONS AND MANAGEMENT

Esophageal manometry is generally a safe procedure; complications are few and typically minor. The most common consequences consist of discomfort, in either the nose or throat, and gagging or retching (**Box 3**). Epistaxis is sometimes encountered, and responds quickly to simple pinching of the nose. If large-volume boluses are administered to patients with oropharyngeal dysphagia or esophageal outflow obstruction, aspiration is a potential risk. Although perforation and transmission of infection are potential complications, they would be considered extremely rare, and have not been formally reported in the literature.

Box 3		
Complications of esophageal manometry		
Common	**Uncommon**	**Rare**
Nasal discomfort	Epistaxis	Infection
Sore throat	Chest pain	Perforation
Gagging	Vasovagal episode	
Retching	Aspiration	

POSTOPERATIVE CARE

When manometry is used to localize the proximal margin of the LES for placement of pH or pH-impedance catheters, placement of these catheters immediately follows the manometry procedure. The operator reads off the distance from the nares to the proximal margin of the LES from the Clouse plots, and inserts the pH or pH-impedance catheter such that the distal tip is 5 cm proximal to the upper border of the LES.

As only topical nasal anesthesia is used, patients can resume their regular diet immediately following removal of the manometry catheter, or following placement of the pH or pH-impedance catheter, as the case may be. Because no sedation is administered, no further postprocedure care is required. The manometry procedure is typically performed on an outpatient basis in most instances, and patients are discharged without the need for a designated driver.

REPORTING, FOLLOW-UP, AND CLINICAL IMPLICATIONS

The pressure data from the HRM study is converted by dedicated software into a color contour plot or Clouse plot, with time on the x-axis, esophageal position on the y-axis (from proximal to distal), and pressure depicted as color contours. Many esophageal motor patterns and abnormalities are visible as distinct patterns on Clouse plots and are readily identified without need for meticulous analysis.[10] Because data are acquired digitally and stored in software programs, computerized interrogation of data is possible with the use of well-tested metrics as described next.[1] Software algorithms have been developed to analyze HRM data according to these accepted metrics, but these computerized analyses need interpretation and oversight to avoid misleading diagnoses, which specifically involve reviewing each test swallow to ensure that anatomic landmarks and measurement parameters are properly identified.[10]

Metrics Used in Clinical HRM Interpretation

IRP consists of 4 continuous or discontinuous seconds of nadir pressure during expected LES relaxation.[5] The IRP is the most important metric used in clinical HRM, as this designates abnormal transit across the LES or EGJ when abnormal. Identification of an abnormal IRP defines the need to resolve esophageal outflow obstruction in a patient with esophageal transit symptoms, such as achalasia. A software tool is used to select the period of expected LES relaxation in determining the IRP. Manual inspection of the swallows determines whether the LES or EGJ remains within the selected IRP assessment box with each swallow, as longitudinal esophageal smooth muscle contraction can sometimes pull the LES proximally away from the assessment box, resulting in a normal IRP and LES pseudorelaxation.

Distal contractile integral (DCI) measures the vigor of esophageal smooth muscle contraction, taking into account the length, amplitude, and duration of contraction, and is reported as mm Hg/cm/s. The DCI is also measured with a software tool, and computed in automated fashion for individual swallows and as a mean of the test swallow complement.[22] The normal mean of 10 swallows has been established as 450 to 5000 mm Hg/cm/s. Individual swallow DCI values higher than 8000 mm Hg/cm/s are never encountered in healthy individuals. Individual swallow values less than 450 mm Hg/cm/s indicate ineffective swallows.

Distal latency (DL) is a measure of timing of peristalsis, measured as the time from UES relaxation to the point where esophageal body peristalsis transitions from fast stripping contraction to slower emptying contraction (termed contractile deceleration point or CDP).[23] Normal DL is greater than 4.5 seconds; when shorter, esophageal stripping cannot occur and sequences are considered premature. Such premature sequences can be seen in the setting of esophageal inhibitory dysfunction.

Peristaltic integrity is assessed using the 20 mm Hg isobaric contour tool, which draws a contour line around pressures at or higher than 20 mm Hg. An intact contour line is seen when peristalsis is intact. Whereas small breaks in the contour line may not necessarily be associated with symptoms, large breaks measuring 5 cm or more designate fragmentation of peristalsis and can be associated with dysphagia and reflux disease.[24]

Reporting Manometry Study Findings

Details included on a manometry study report are described in **Box 4**. A manometry report includes patient demographics and the indication for the study. The latter is particularly important, as interpretation and clinical opinions need to relate to the symptoms being investigated and the clinical question being asked in evaluating esophageal motor function. When studies are performed by a trained nurse or technician, it is important that patient symptoms are extracted from records, direct patient interview, or patient questionnaires.

The report describes resting characteristics of the UES and LES during the landmark phase. The UES and LES are seen as horizontal bands of higher-pressure color, with variations in pressure induced by respiration as cyclical changes in color. Separation between the LES and diaphragmatic crura constitutes a hiatus hernia. Anatomic measurements including locations of the UES and LES, esophageal length, and length of hiatus hernia are reported.

Next, the impact of test swallows on esophageal motor function are reported, using normative values developed specifically for the particular type of catheter used, as normative values can vary between catheter types made by different manufacturers.[25] In assessing test swallows, peristaltic performance is reported as

---

Box 4
Components of a manometry report

- Demographics

- Indication for the study

- Anatomic parameters: esophageal length, location of upper esophageal sphincter (UES) and lower esophageal sphincter (LES), hiatus hernia, pressure inversion point

- Peristaltic performance: proportions of peristaltic, premature, and failed sequences

- LES parameters: basal resting LES pressure, end expiratory LES pressure, residual pressure (integrated relaxation pressure)

- UES parameters: basal UES pressure, postswallow residual pressure

- Esophageal body parameters: distal contractile integral, distal latency, peristaltic integrity (intact peristalsis, breaks >5 cm in the peristaltic contour)

- Alternative swallow position metrics, interpretation

- Alternative bolus consistency metrics, interpretation

- Provocative measures, interpretation

- Bolus transit (when impedance is combined with manometry)

- Final diagnosis based on Chicago Classification

- Interpretation of symptoms and clinical implications

proportions of peristaltic, premature, and failed swallows. Sphincter relaxation during test swallows is reported, particularly LES relaxation, designated as the mean IRP. Esophageal body metrics are reported in terms of DCI and DL. It is important to add a descriptive element, reporting contraction wave abnormalities, breaks in the peristaltic contour, and proximal skeletal muscle contraction, as minor abnormalities in motor function may be lost during the averaging process of deriving HRM metrics. Use of HRM metrics in designating motor diagnoses is described elsewhere in this issue.

Finally, findings on alternative swallow positions (eg, upright swallows), alternative test boluses (viscous, solid), and results of provocative testing are described. The implications of these findings on eventual diagnosis may require further interpretation and description in the final report.

Follow-Up

Esophageal manometry comprises only 1 component of esophageal function testing, and information obtained from esophageal manometry needs to be interpreted in the context of patient symptoms and results on complementary tests. Upper endoscopy and barium contrast studies are frequently used in conjunction with esophageal manometry, particularly in identifying mucosal inflammatory processes, obtaining anatomic details, or diagnosing structural restrictive processes in the esophagus.[1] Endoscopic ultrasonography is increasingly being used to rule out infiltrative processes at the EGJ, especially when esophageal outflow obstruction is identified. Impedance planimetry or a functional luminal imaging probe can provide further information on esophageal and EGJ compliance.

Clinical Implications

The finding of an abnormally high IRP indicates abnormal transit across the LES or EGJ, and requires some form of management directed at improving transit across the EGJ in the presence of compatible symptoms. Although abnormal IRP characterizes achalasia when esophageal body peristalsis is absent or premature, this finding prompts further evaluation for structural or infiltrative processes in the setting of atypical features. When achalasia is diagnosed, subtyping based on presence or absence of pressurization and premature contractions helps predict treatment outcome, as described by Pandolfino and colleagues.[26] At the other end of the spectrum, a structurally deficient EGJ (hypotensive LES, presence of a hiatus hernia) may predict significant gastroesophageal reflux that sometimes triggers surgical repair.

Clinical implications of absent or severely compromised esophageal body peristalsis relate to abnormal bolus transit, resulting in transit symptoms such as dysphagia, and abnormal reflux clearance resulting in prolonged acid exposure times. A standard 360° fundoplication may result in dysphagia, and only a 270° partial fundoplication is possible in these circumstances. Lesser degrees of hypomotility may manifest as varying proportions of ineffective peristalsis[27]; in these instances, provocative testing may identify peristaltic reserve when esophageal body contraction normalizes following the provocative maneuver.[18]

Exaggerated esophageal body peristalsis may be associated with perceptive symptoms such as chest pain, and sometimes transit symptoms such as dysphagia. Clinical implications depend on the dominant symptom being investigated: perceptive symptoms may improve with neuromodulators and treatment of noxious triggers such as reflux, whereas transit symptoms may require smooth-muscle relaxants or measures to disrupt smooth-muscle contraction (eg, extended myotomy).

OUTCOMES
Reproducibility

When HRM studies were repeated on 2 consecutive days in 20 healthy volunteers, concordance was high for anatomic parameters such as UES basal pressure, transition-zone length, LES basal pressure, LES postswallow residual pressure, and distal esophageal contraction amplitude. There was intermediate concordance for parameters of function, such as DCI, IRP, and proximal contraction amplitude, which varied swallow-to-swallow and day-to-day, but the overall pattern did not seem to significantly change.[28] Inherent variations in motor contraction parameters have been recognized to occur between swallows in healthy controls and patients with esophageal symptoms, and may be partly related to swallow volume and refractory state of esophageal smooth muscle following swallows.[29] The clinical significance of some of these variations can be further addressed with provocative testing. HRM therefore has good reproducibility under standard test conditions.

Comprehension and Retention

The image-based paradigm of HRM lends itself well to comprehension of esophageal motor function. After a short tutorial, novice and intermediate learners of esophageal physiology and pathophysiology (medical students, internal medicine residents, and gastroenterology fellows) consistently preferred HRM to conventional line tracings. On assessment of diagnostic accuracy for broad groups of esophageal motor disorders immediately after the tutorial and again 4 months later, there were consistent gains with HRM over conventional line tracings at both data points.[30] Others have demonstrated similar benefits from the spatiotemporal Clouse plot,[31] which lends itself to pattern recognition, especially of well-developed motor patterns such as achalasia and aperistalsis.

CURRENT CONTROVERSIES
Artifacts

Equipment-related artifacts

Because the HRM catheter is pressure calibrated at room temperature but pressure acquisition is performed at body temperature, there can be differences in recorded and reported pressures with a median temperature difference (or thermal effect) of 7 mm Hg.[7] Two measures can help in correcting this discrepancy. First, a compensation factor can be obtained by immersing the HRM catheter in a water bath at body temperature (37°C at 2-cm depth). Second, a thermal compensation maneuver can be performed after each study, whereby the catheter is held up in mid-air after extubation and the thermal compensation software algorithm tool is used with the cursor positioned during this period of the recording.

An issue with prolonged studies of greater than 20 to 30 minutes in duration is that recorded pressures are susceptible to thermal drift. This drift is linear and only partially corrected by the thermal compensation maneuver. Instead, a linear correction may need to be applied for prolonged HRM studies to more fully correct for this phenomenon.[7]

Electronic equipment may be subject to malfunction, especially if leaks are present in the catheter and bodily fluids or cleansing solution get into the catheter assembly. Unusual pressure differentials may be seen throughout the recording at one unique level. If only 1 noncritical sensor malfunctions, it can be turned off using a menu function, and the software algorithm will then average pressures from the adjacent 2 sensors to retain a smooth contour in the Clouse plot. If the location of the aberrant sensor is across a sphincter, recorded pressures and metrics may not be accurate, and the HRM catheter will likely require servicing or replacement.

Vascular and respiratory artifacts

Interpretation may be affected by prominent artifacts from other structures, especially the heart.[32] Two levels of cardiac impression are typically seen, one in the mid-esophagus from the aortic arch and another more distally from the left atrium. Respiratory artifacts can consist of alternating bands of pressure to coincide with the respiratory cycle, especially in patients with tachypnea or obstructive pulmonary disease. When vigorous respiration coincides with the peristaltic sequence, artifacts can be generated that can suggest repetitive contraction of esophageal smooth muscle.[33] Cardiac artifacts may be reduced by asking patients to tilt slightly to the left while supine, allowing the cardiac structures to fall away from the esophagus (**Fig. 6**). Respiratory artifacts are more difficult to resolve, but patients can be allowed to relax, which can reduce respiratory rate.

FUTURE CONSIDERATIONS
High-Resolution Impedance Manometry

Modern manometry catheters have the option of embedding impedance rings between pressure sensors, which allows assessment of bolus transit concurrent with pressure measurement. Typically, saline boluses are used in such studies to allow better visibility on impedance contour plots. High-resolution impedance manometry (HRIM) has been used to determine the effectiveness of peristalsis in relation to bolus transit.[1] Using this technology, bolus transit has been demonstrated to be complete with contraction amplitudes as low as 20 mm Hg, as long as no large breaks (>5 cm) exist in the peristaltic contour.[34] The clinical utility of this technology in predicting symptoms or in directing patient management beyond information that can routinely be obtained from HRM alone continues to be evaluated. One area wherein HRIM has demonstrated clinical usefulness is in predicting bolus transit across the EGJ following therapy for achalasia. The column of water in the esophagus 5 minutes after a 200-mL water challenge has been demonstrated to correlate well with the barium column at a similar time frame on a timed upright barium study in patients with achalasia, suggesting that HRIM could replace timed upright barium studies in evaluating the efficacy of LES disruption in achalasia.[35]

Three-Dimensional Manometry

Increased sensor density over a distal 9-cm segment on an HRM catheter allows mapping of the 3-dimensional structure of both sphincters (UES and LES) and the EGJ.[36,37] This technology has been used successfully in the assessment of anorectal sphincter morphology and physiology. Such 3-dimensional mapping may provide

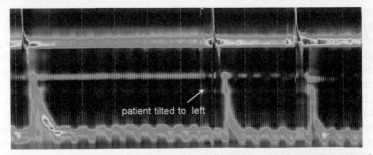

patient tilted to left

Fig. 6. Vascular artifact, seen as a band of pressure fluctuating at the same rate as the pulse. The patient was tilted slightly to the left, which allowed the heart to shift away from the esophagus. This action resolved the artifact.

more detailed assessment of LES relaxation and EGJ morphology, although it is unclear whether this additional information translates into better clinical utility. Further research is needed.

SUMMARY

HRM represents a significant advance in esophageal function testing. Real-time images allow accurate identification of esophageal landmarks by the operator, eliminating the stationary pull-through maneuver and shortening the duration of the manometry procedure. Abnormal LES relaxation is diagnosed with high accuracy. Supine wet swallows continue to be used for standard analysis, but upright swallows and provocative maneuvers may augment recognition of motor processes. Although automated analysis using software tools has improved interpretation, the operator needs to oversee accurate depiction of landmarks and peristaltic parameters. The incorporation of impedance technology allows bolus visualization, and increased sensor density (3-dimensional manometry) has the potential to improve the evaluation of sphincter function under certain circumstances.

REFERENCES

1. Gyawali CP, Bredenoord AJ, Conklin JL, et al. Evaluation of esophageal motor function in clinical practice. Neurogastroenterol Motil 2013;25:99–133.
2. Clouse RE, Prakash C. Topographic esophageal manometry: an emerging clinical and investigative approach. Dig Dis 2000;18:64–74.
3. Kahrilas PJ. Esophageal motor disorders in terms of high-resolution esophageal pressure topography: what has changed? Am J Gastroenterol 2010;105:981–7.
4. Gyawali CP. High resolution manometry: the Ray Clouse legacy. Neurogastroenterol Motil 2012;24(Suppl 1):2–4.
5. Ghosh SK, Pandolfino JE, Rice J, et al. Impaired deglutitive EGJ relaxation in clinical esophageal manometry: a quantitative analysis of 400 patients and 75 controls. Am J Physiol Gastrointest Liver Physiol 2007;293:G878–85.
6. Murray JA, Clouse RE, Conklin JL. Components of the standard oesophageal manometry. Neurogastroenterol Motil 2003;15:591–606.
7. Robertson EV, Lee YY, Derakhshan MH, et al. High-resolution esophageal manometry: addressing thermal drift of the manoscan system. Neurogastroenterol Motil 2012;24:61–4, e11.
8. Gyawali CP, Bredenoord AJ, Conklin JL, et al. Esophageal high resolution manometry in a community practice. Neurogastroenterol Motil 2013;25:776–7.
9. Gyawali CP. Making the most of imperfect high-resolution manometry studies. Clin Gastroenterol Hepatol 2011;9:1015–6.
10. Conklin JL. Evaluation of esophageal motor function with high-resolution manometry. J Neurogastroenterol Motil 2013;19:281–94.
11. Sweis R, Anggiansah A, Wong T, et al. Normative values and inter-observer agreement for liquid and solid bolus swallows in upright and supine positions as assessed by esophageal high-resolution manometry. Neurogastroenterol Motil 2011;23:509–e198.
12. Roman S, Damon H, Pellissier PE, et al. Does body position modify the results of oesophageal high resolution manometry? Neurogastroenterol Motil 2010;22:271–5.
13. Roman S, Kahrilas PJ, Boris L, et al. High-resolution manometry studies are frequently imperfect but usually still interpretable. Clin Gastroenterol Hepatol 2011;9:1050–5.

14. Patel A, Mirza F, Gyawali CP. Optimizing the high resolution manometry (HRM) study protocol. Gastroenterology 2013;144:S-263.
15. Sifrim D, Janssens J, Vantrappen G. A wave of inhibition precedes primary peristaltic contractions in the human esophagus. Gastroenterology 1992;103:876–82.
16. Bredenoord AJ, Fox M, Kahrilas PJ, et al. Chicago classification criteria of esophageal motility disorders defined in high resolution esophageal pressure topography. Neurogastroenterol Motil 2012;24(Suppl 1):57–65.
17. Xiao Y, Nicodeme F, Kahrilas PJ, et al. Optimizing the swallow protocol of clinical high-resolution esophageal manometry studies. Neurogastroenterol Motil 2012; 24:e489–96.
18. Shaker A, Stoikes N, Drapekin J, et al. Multiple rapid swallow responses during esophageal high-resolution manometry reflect esophageal body peristaltic reserve. Am J Gastroenterol 2013;108:1706–12.
19. Stoikes N, Drapekin J, Kushnir V, et al. The value of multiple rapid swallows during preoperative esophageal manometry before laparoscopic antireflux surgery. Surg Endosc 2012;26:3401–7.
20. Kushnir V, Sayuk GS, Gyawali CP. Multiple rapid swallow responses segregate achalasia subtypes on high-resolution manometry. Neurogastroenterol Motil 2012;24:1069-e561.
21. Pouderoux P, Shi G, Tatum RP, et al. Esophageal solid bolus transit: studies using concurrent videofluoroscopy and manometry. Am J Gastroenterol 1999;94: 1457–63.
22. Ghosh SK, Pandolfino JE, Zhang Q, et al. Quantifying esophageal peristalsis with high-resolution manometry: a study of 75 asymptomatic volunteers. Am J Physiol Gastrointest Liver Physiol 2006;290:G988–97.
23. Roman S, Lin Z, Pandolfino JE, et al. Distal contraction latency: a measure of propagation velocity optimized for esophageal pressure topography studies. Am J Gastroenterol 2011;106:443–51.
24. Porter RF, Kumar N, Drapekin JE, et al. Fragmented esophageal smooth muscle contraction segments on high resolution manometry: a marker of esophageal hypomotility. Neurogastroenterol Motil 2012;24:763–8, e353.
25. Bogte A, Bredenoord AJ, Oors J, et al. Normal values for esophageal high-resolution manometry. Neurogastroenterol Motil 2013;25:762-e579.
26. Pandolfino JE, Kwiatek MA, Nealis T, et al. Achalasia: a new clinically relevant classification by high-resolution manometry. Gastroenterology 2008;135:1526–33.
27. Xiao Y, Kahrilas PJ, Kwasny MJ, et al. High-resolution manometry correlates of ineffective esophageal motility. Am J Gastroenterol 2012;107:1647–54.
28. Bogte A, Bredenoord AJ, Oors J, et al. Reproducibility of esophageal high-resolution manometry. Neurogastroenterol Motil 2011;23:e271–6.
29. Clouse RE, Alrakawi A, Staiano A. Intersubject and interswallow variability in topography of esophageal motility. Dig Dis Sci 1998;43:1978–85.
30. Soudagar AS, Sayuk GS, Gyawali CP. Learners favour high resolution oesophageal manometry with better diagnostic accuracy over conventional line tracings. Gut 2012;61:798–803.
31. Grubel C, Hiscock R, Hebbard G. Value of spatiotemporal representation of manometric data. Clin Gastroenterol Hepatol 2008;6:525–30.
32. Babaei A, Mittal RK. Cardiovascular compression of the esophagus and spread of gastro-esophageal reflux. Neurogastroenterol Motil 2011;23:45–51, e3.
33. Sampath NJ, Bhargava V, Mittal RK. Genesis of multipeaked waves of the esophagus: repetitive contractions or motion artifact? Am J Physiol Gastrointest Liver Physiol 2010;298:G927–33.

34. Roman S, Lin Z, Kwiatek MA, et al. Weak peristalsis in esophageal pressure topography: classification and association with dysphagia. Am J Gastroenterol 2011;106:349–56.
35. Cho YK, Lipowska AM, Nicodeme F, et al. Assessing bolus retention in achalasia using high-resolution manometry with impedance: a comparator study with timed barium esophagram. Am J Gastroenterol 2014;109(6):829–35.
36. Kwiatek MA, Pandolfino JE, Kahrilas PJ. 3D-high resolution manometry of the esophagogastric junction. Neurogastroenterol Motil 2011;23:e461–9.
37. Nicodeme F, Lin Z, Pandolfino JE, et al. Esophagogastric junction pressure morphology: comparison between a station pull-through and real-time 3D-HRM representation. Neurogastroenterol Motil 2013;25:e591–8.

The Chicago Classification of Motility Disorders
An Update

Sabine Roman, MD, PhD[a], C. Prakash Gyawali, MD, MRCP[b],
Yinglian Xiao, MD, PhD[c], John E. Pandolfino, MD, MSci[d],
Peter J. Kahrilas, MD[d],*

KEYWORDS

- Esophageal high-resolution manometry • Achalasia
- Esophagogastric junction outflow obstruction • Aperistalsis
- Distal esophageal spasm • Hypercontractile esophagus
- Ineffective esophageal motility

KEY POINTS

- The Chicago Classification of esophageal motility disorders is based on a clinical study comprising 10 test swallows performed in a supine posture.
- Esophageal motility disorders are divided into disorders with esophagogastric junction outflow obstruction, major disorders not encountered in normal subjects, and minor motility disorders defined by statistical abnormalities.
- Three subtypes of achalasia are defined that are clinically distinct in terms of responsiveness to therapeutic intervention.
- Major esophageal motility disorders are aperistalsis, distal esophageal spasm, and hypercontractile (jackhammer) esophagus.
- Ineffective esophageal motility is likely to replace weak peristalsis and frequent peristalsis in version 3.0 of the Chicago Classification.

This work was supported by grant no. R01 DK079902 (J.E. Pandolfino) and R01 DK56033 (P.J. Kahrilas) from the National Institutes of Health.
Conflict of Interest: S. Roman has served as consultant for Given Imaging.
[a] Digestive Physiology, Hôpital E Herriot, Hospices Civils de Lyon, Claude Bernard Lyon I University, Pavillon H, 5 Place d'Arsonval, Cedex 03, Lyon F-69437, France; [b] Division of Gastroenterology, Washington University School of Medicine, 660 South Euclid Avenue, Campus Box 8124, St Louis, MO 63110, USA; [c] Department of Gastroenterology and Hepatology, The First Affiliated Hospital, Sun Yat-sen University, 58 Zhongshan Road 2, Guangzhou 510080, China; [d] Department of Medicine, Feinberg School of Medicine, Northwestern University, 676 St Clair Street, 14th Floor, Chicago, IL 60611-2951, USA
* Corresponding author.
E-mail address: p-kahrilas@northwestern.edu

Gastrointest Endoscopy Clin N Am 24 (2014) 545–561
http://dx.doi.org/10.1016/j.giec.2014.07.001
1052-5157/14/$ – see front matter © 2014 Elsevier Inc. All rights reserved.
giendo.theclinics.com

INTRODUCTION

High-resolution manometry (HRM) is the current gold standard technique to assess esophageal motility. It uses closely spaced pressure sensors to create a dynamic representation of pressure change along the entire length of the esophagus. Data acquisition is easier than with conventional manometry and interpretation is facilitated by esophageal pressure topography (Clouse) plots.[1]

Along with the technological innovation, an international consensus process has evolved over recent years to define esophageal motility disorders using HRM, Clouse plots, and standardized metrics. This classification, titled the Chicago Classification, was firstly published in 2009[2] and was subsequently updated in 2012.[3] It was intended to be applied to HRM studies performed in a supine position with 5-mL water swallows and for patients without previous esophagogastric surgery. The 2012 version of the Chicago Classification focused entirely on redefining esophageal motor disorders associated with dysphagia in HRM terms; it did not provide guidance on the assessment of the esophagogastric junction (EGJ) at rest or upper esophageal sphincter (UES) function. Since that publication, substantial further research has been presented and published, intended to improve the diagnostic accuracy and clinical utility of the Chicago Classification. In recognition of this, the international HRM Working Group met in Chicago in May 2014 in conjunction with Digestive Disease Week to discuss these new data in the context of working toward an update of the Chicago Classification (v3.0). This article presents a brief summary of these discussions and proposals to work toward the Chicago Classification 3.0; a process due to be completed in early 2015.

METRICS AND SWALLOW PATTERN CHARACTERIZATION

The Chicago Classification is based on scoring of 10 5-mL water swallows performed in supine position. EGJ relaxation, esophageal contractile activity, and esophageal pressurization are evaluated for each swallow. However, a major indication for manometric studies is in the evaluation of patients for potential antireflux surgery and some description of EGJ morphology and quantification of contractility is desirable. Hence, the incorporation of simple metrics relevant to these aspects of motility will be incorporated into Chicago Classification v3.0. Proposed metrics under discussion include mean inspiratory pressure, mean expiratory pressure, the extent and variability of the separation between the lower esophageal sphincter (LES) and crural diaphragm (CD separation), and the EGJ contractile integral (CI), all of which have been used in publications. However, discrepancies exist in the details of calculation methodology for these metrics, the strength of data supporting their utility, and their normative ranges among HRM devices,[4–11] all of which are important limitations meriting further consideration.

Esophagogastric Junction Morphology and Deglutitive Relaxation

With HRM and Clouse plots, the relative localization of the 2 constituents of the EGJ, the LES and the CD, define EGJ morphologic subtypes.[12] This feature of EGJ morphology is fundamental, and is likely pertinent to its functional integrity. With type I EGJ morphology, there is complete overlap of the CD and LES with no spatial separation evident on the Clouse plot (**Fig. 1**) and no double peak on the associated spatial pressure variation plot. With type II EGJ morphology, the LES and CD are separated (double-peaked spatial pressure variation plot), but the nadir pressure between the 2 peaks does not decline to gastric pressure; the separation between the pressure peaks is less than 3 cm. With type III EGJ morphology, the LES and CD are clearly

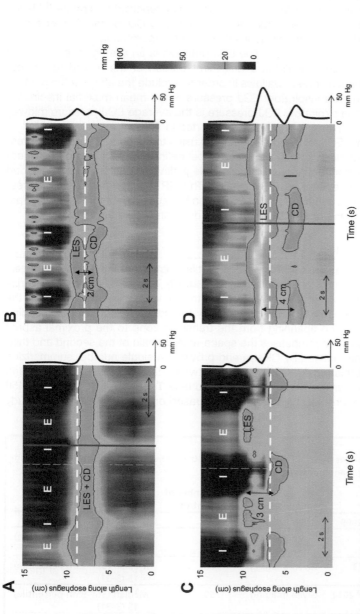

Fig. 1. EGJ morphology subtypes. For each panel the instantaneous spatial pressure variation plot corresponding with the red line on the pressure topography plot is shown by the black line on the right. The 2 main EGJ components are the LES and the CD, which cannot be independently quantified when they are superimposed, as with a type I EGJ (*A*). The respiratory inversion point (RIP), shown by the horizontal dashed line, is at the proximal margin of the EGJ. During inspiration (I), EGJ pressure increases, whereas it decreases during expiration (E). Type II EGJ pressure morphology is shown in (*B*). Note the 2 peaks on the instantaneous spatial pressure variation plot; the nadir pressure between the peaks is greater than the intragastric pressure. (*C, D*) Type III EGJ pressure morphology defined as the presence of 2 peaks of the instantaneous spatial pressure variation plot with a nadir pressure between the peaks equal to or less than intragastric pressure. The RIP is proximal to the CD with type IIIa (*C*), whereas it is proximal to the LES in IIIb (*D*).

separated as shown by a double-peaked spatial pressure variation plot and a nadir pressure between the peaks equal to or less than gastric pressure; with type IIIa the pressure inversion point remains at the CD level, whereas in type IIIb it is located at the LES level. However, the separation between LES and CD may fluctuate in the course of the study and in those instances this should be reported as a range.[13] Hence in reporting the LES-CD, the range of observed LES-CD separation observed throughout the study is reported for types II and III EGJ morphology.

The simplest measurement of baseline EGJ pressure is an average pressure for 3 normal respiratory cycles, ideally in a quiescent portion of the recording, remote from either spontaneous or test swallows in order to exclude the effect of the postdeglutitive contraction. The inspiratory EGJ pressure is the mean maximal inspiratory EGJ pressure and the expiratory EGJ pressure is the average EGJ pressure midway between inspirations. Normative values are reported in **Table 1**.

During swallowing, EGJ relaxation is evaluated using the integrated relaxation pressure (IRP), which has been (and will continue to be) defined as the mean of the 4 seconds (contiguous or noncontiguous) of maximal deglutitive relaxation in the 10-second window beginning at deglutitive UES relaxation. The IRP is referenced to gastric pressure. However, normal values depend strongly on the specific manometric hardware used, making this an important diagnostic consideration (**Table 2**).

Deglutitive Peristaltic Vigor and Pattern

Metrics are used to evaluate esophageal contractile function are the distal esophageal integral (DCI) and the distal latency (DL) (**Fig. 2**, **Table 3**). They are used to characterize each of the 10 5-mL test swallows (**Table 4**). Contractile vigor is summarized using the DCI. This metric applies an algorithm to quantify the contractile pressure exceeding 20 mm Hg for the region spanning from the transition zone to the proximal aspect of the EGJ. As such, it encompasses the space-time domain of the second and third contractile segments defined by Clouse and provides a single number summarizing contractile vigor in this region. Cutoff values between diagnostic categories depend on the manometric hardware and software used (see **Table 3**). A DCI between 450 and 8000 mm Hg·s·cm is considered normal. Based on the conclusions of a study

Table 1
Reported normal ranges of basal EGJ pressures for control subjects in a supine position among studies and among manometric devices

Author	Equipment	Number of Controls	End-expiratory EGJ Pressure (mm Hg)
Pandolfino et al,[2] 2009	Given Imaging	75	Mean (±2 SD) = 18 (4–33)
Sweis et al,[9] 2011	Given Imaging	23	Median (5th–95th percentile) 19 (5–38)
Niebisch et al,[8] 2013	Given Imaging	68	Median (5th–95th percentile) 15 (3–31)
Weijenborg et al,[10] 2014	Given Imaging	50	Median (5th–95th percentile) 15 (3–31)
Bogte et al,[4] 2013	MMS (solid state; Unisensor AG)	52	Median (5th–95th percentile) 31 (9–51)
Kessing et al,[7] 2014	MMS (water-perfused system)	50	Median (5th–95th percentile) 10 (3–30)

Abbreviation: MMS, medical measurement systems; SD, standard deviation.

Table 2
Reported normal ranges of IRP for control subjects in a supine position among studies and among manometric devices

Author	Equipment	Number of Controls	IRP (mm Hg) 95th Percentile = ULN	
			Mean	Median (ULN)
Ghosh et al,[5] 2007	Given Imaging	75	9	8 (15)
Sweis et al,[9] 2011	Given Imaging	23	4	3 (9)
Niebisch et al,[8] 2013	Given Imaging	68	9	9 (17)
Weijenborg et al,[10] 2014	Given Imaging	50	8	7 (16)
Bogte et al,[4] 2013	MMS (solid state; Unisensor AG)	52	13	12 (28)
Kessing et al,[7] 2014	MMS (water-perfused system)	50	8	7 (19)

Abbreviation: ULN, upper limit of normal.

on ineffective contractile contraction,[14] the international HRM Working Group is inclined to define failed and weak contraction based on the DCI value in the Chicago Classification v3.0. The current proposal is that a contraction with a DCI less than 100 mm Hg·s·cm defines a failed contraction and a weak contraction is defined as

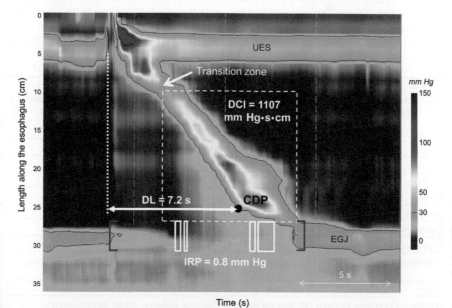

Time (s)

Fig. 2. Normal esophageal peristaltic contraction. The IRP is measured during the deglutitive window, indicated by the brown bracket. The IRP is the lowest pressure for 4 seconds (contiguous or noncontiguous), identified by the white boxes within the deglutitive window. The distal contractile integral (DCI) is measured from the transition zone to the EGJ, equating to the product of the amplitude times the duration times the length of the contraction located within the dashed box. The contractile deceleration point (CDP; *black dot*) represents the inflexion point in the velocity of contractile front propagation. DL is measured from UES relaxation (*dashed vertical line*) to the CDP.

Table 3
Reported normal ranges of distal contractile integral (DCI) and DL for control subjects in a supine position among studies and among manometric devices

Author	Equipment	Number of Controls	Median DCI (5th–95th Percentile) (mm Hg·s·cm)	Median DL (5th Percentile) (s)
Xiao et al,[11] 2012	Given Imaging	75	1612 (448–4721)	5.8 (4.3)
Niebisch et al,[8] 2013	Given Imaging	68	1485 (420–4236)	6.8 (5.4)
Weijenborg et al,[10] 2014	Given Imaging	50	834 (178–2828)	6.8 (5.4)
Bogte et al,[4] 2013	MMS (solid state; Unisensor AG)	52	1008 (186–3407)	6.1 (5.0)
Kessing et al,[7] 2014	MMS (water-perfused system)	50	970 (142–3675)	7.4 (6.2)

a DCI greater than 100 mm Hg·s·cm but less than 450 mm Hg·s·cm. Both failed and weak contractions are ineffective. In addition, a DCI greater than or equal to 8000 mm Hg·s·cm defines hypercontractility.[15]

The contractile deceleration point (CDP) is a key landmark in the assessment of the contraction pattern. It represents the inflexion point in the contractile front propagation velocity on the 30 mm Hg isobaric contour in the distal esophagus.[16] After the CDP, propagation velocity slows, signifying the termination of peristalsis and the onset of ampullary emptying; this is usually located 2 to 3 cm proximal to the EGJ.[17] The DL

Table 4
Characteristics of deglutitive peristaltic function proposed for the Chicago Classification v3.0 (note that contraction pattern is not scored with failed or weak vigor)

Contractile Vigor	
Failed	DCI <100 mm Hg·s·cm
Weak	DCI >100 mm Hg·s·cm, but <450 mm Hg·s·cm
Ineffective	Failed or weak
Normal	DCI >450 mm Hg·s·cm but <8000 mm Hg·s·cm
Hypercontractile	DCI ≥8000 mm Hg·s·cm
Contraction Pattern	
Premature	DL <4.5 s
Fragmented	Large break (>5 cm) in the 20 mm Hg isobaric contour, but not failed and DCI >450 mm Hg·s·cm
Intact	Not achieving the diagnostic criteria listed earlier
Intrabolus Pressure Pattern (30 mm Hg Isobaric Contour Referenced to Atmospheric)	
Panesophageal pressurization	Uniform pressurization of >30 mm Hg extending from the UES to the EGJ
Compartmentalized esophageal pressurization	Pressurization of >30 mm Hg extending from the contractile front to the EGJ
EGJ pressurization	Pressurization restricted to zone between the LES and CD in conjunction with LES-CD separation
Normal	No bolus pressurization >30 mm Hg

corresponds with the period of deglutitive inhibition that precedes esophageal contraction at the CDP and it is measured as the interval from UES relaxation to the CDP.[18] A value less than 4.5 seconds is considered abnormal and defines a premature contraction. However, if the contraction is weak (DCI <450 mm Hg·s·cm) with a DL less than 4.5 seconds, it may be considered a failed contraction because this contraction is most likely ineffective (**Fig. 3**D).

The contractile front velocity (CFV) is estimated by determining the slope of the tangent skirting the 30 mm Hg isobaric contour from the transition zone to the CDP. Although this metric of velocity has historical relevance, it has been removed from the Chicago Classification v3.0 because of its lack of specificity to define esophageal spasm and the unknown clinical relevance of rapid contraction with normal DL.

Peristaltic integrity is defined by gaps in the 20 mm Hg isobaric contour of the peristaltic contraction between the UES and EGJ. Although no longer used in defining weak peristalsis, peristaltic integrity is still proposed as an important morphologic characteristic of peristalsis in Chicago Classification v3.0 (**Fig. 4**D). Although the 2012 classification distinguished small (2–5 cm in length) and large (>5 cm) breaks as subtypes of weak peristalsis, the Working Group proposes that small breaks be considered normal and that only breaks greater than 5 cm in length be scored. In addition, the nomenclature has changed to distinguish between contractions with breaks

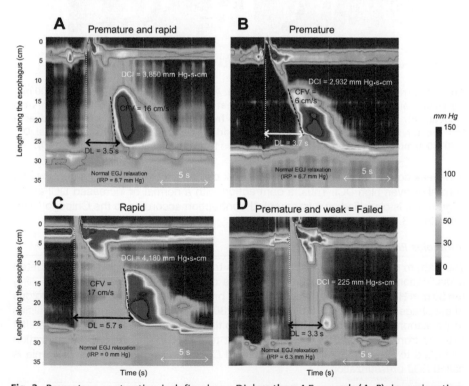

Fig. 3. Premature contraction is defined as a DL less than 4.5 seconds (*A, B*); in conjunction with normal EGJ relaxation they are the defining features of distal esophageal spasm. The contractile front velocity (CFV) of a premature contraction might be increased (>9 cm/s) (*A*) or normal (*B*). The clinical significance of rapid contraction with normal DL (*C*) remains to be determined. A weak contraction (DCI <450 mm Hg·s·cm) with a reduced DL is considered failed (*D*).

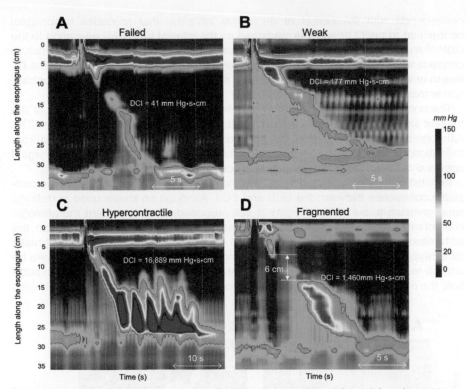

Fig. 4. Contractile vigor is assessed using the DCI. A contraction with a DCI less than 100 mm Hg·s·cm is failed (*A*). A contraction with a DCI greater than 100 but less than 450 mm Hg·s·cm is weak (*B*). Both are ineffective swallows. A hypercontractile swallow is defined as a DCI greater than 8000 mm Hg·s·cm (*C*). In addition, a contraction with a normal DCI (450–8000 mm Hg·s·cm) and a break greater than 5 cm is a fragmented contraction (*D*).

and weak contractions because a large break can be encountered in the context of a normal or even high DCI. Thus, a contraction with a normal or increased DCI and a large break is classified as a fragmented contraction according to the Chicago Classification v3.0.

Intrabolus Pressure Pattern

The pattern of intrabolus pressure continues to be an important part of the updated classification scheme. Intrabolus pressure is characterized for each swallow using the 30 mm Hg isobaric contour and abnormal pressurization corresponds with regions of esophageal pressurization to greater than 30 mm Hg. Intrabolus pressure qualifies as panesophageal if it spans from the EGJ to the UES and as compartmentalized if it extends from the deglutitive contractile front to the EGJ. In addition, pressurization restricted to the zone between the LES and CD in conjunction with hiatal hernia is called EGJ pressurization.

DISORDERS WITH EGJ OUTFLOW OBSTRUCTION

The most fundamental assessment of deglutitive contractility in the Chicago Classification is of whether or not an EGJ outflow obstruction is present as defined by the IRP. Disorders of EGJ outflow obstruction are further subdivided into achalasia subtypes and EGJ outflow obstruction based on the contractile and pressurization patterns in the body of the esophagus (**Fig. 5**). Three clinically relevant subtypes of achalasia have been defined in the previous iteration of the Chicago Classification.[19] Type I achalasia was characterized by 100% failed contractions and no esophageal pressurization, type II achalasia was defined as 100% failed contraction and panesophageal pressurization for at least 20% of swallows, and type III achalasia was defined as the presence of preserved fragments of distal peristalsis or premature contractions for at least 20% of the swallows in the 2012 Chicago Classification.

The international HRM Working Group had several suggestions to improve and clarify these definitions in the Chicago Classification v3.0. First, the Working Group proposed that it is more relevant to base the evaluation of EGJ relaxation on the median rather than the mean IRP of 10 swallows in order to minimize the effect of occasional outliers that occur for a variety of reasons. Second, using a classification and regression tree (CART) model, it has recently been shown that the critical IRP threshold may vary among achalasia subtypes.[20] In type I achalasia, IRP threshold might be reduced to a cutoff value as low as 10 mm Hg to more accurately distinguish it from aperistalsis. Third, the occurrence of panesophageal pressurization for at least 20% of swallows in conjunction with 100% failed contractions diagnoses type II

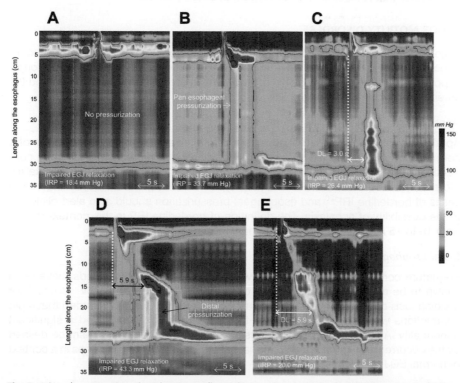

Fig. 5. Disorders associated with EGJ outflow obstruction. Impaired EGJ relaxation is evident from an IRP greater than 15 mm Hg. In type I achalasia there is no esophageal contraction and no esophageal pressurization (*A*). Type II achalasia is characterized by panesophageal pressurization and absence of a peristaltic contraction (*B*). In type III achalasia, there is at least 20% premature contraction, defined as DL less than 4.5 seconds (*C*). EGJ outflow obstruction may represent a variant of achalasia (*D*). It might also be the consequence of a mechanical obstruction (*E*) such as a distal esophageal stenosis in a context of esophagitis.

achalasia regardless of the IRP value. Fourth, it was acknowledged that the critical IRP cutoff varied among manometric devices (see **Table 2**). However, in order to simplify the use of the Chicago Classification v3.0 in clinical practice, the current thinking of the HRM Working Group is that it is better to keep the same IRP threshold for all achalasia subtypes but leave some flexibility in interpretation when certain combinations of contractility are observed. For instance, because of the relevance of this regression tree model analysis, the HRM Working Group suggested the addition of a qualifier to the diagnosis of aperistalsis (discussed later): in instances of 100% failed contractions, a diagnosis of achalasia should be considered if there is a borderline median IRP value or if there is evidence of esophageal pressurization.

Another observation that is relevant to contractile features defining type III achalasia is that after pneumatic dilation or, more commonly, Heller myotomy, instances of peristalsis can be observed that were not observed before treatment.[21] This observation led to the hypothesis that esophageal pressurization might have hidden some instances of peristalsis in the pretreatment studies. Hence, the Working Group proposed that, in Chicago Classification v3.0, the definition of type III achalasia should be restricted to premature contractions. In addition, EGJ outflow obstruction is characterized by an increased median IRP associated with evidence of esophageal contractility that is inconsistent with type I, II, or III achalasia.

MAJOR MOTILITY DISORDERS

Major motility disorders are defined as patterns of motor function that are not encountered in controls in the context of normal EGJ relaxation. The Working Group strongly supported the continued use of this criterion but, in some cases, slightly modified the criteria for defining the major motility disorders (**Table 5**).

Aperistalsis

Aperistalsis (previously called absent peristalsis) is defined by the combination of a normal IRP and 100% failed contractions. As mentioned previously, premature contractions with DCI less than 100 mm Hg·s·cm meet the criteria for failed peristalsis. Moreover, based on the CART analysis, type I achalasia should be considered in cases of borderline IRP[20] and esophageal pressurization should also alert clinicians to the possibility of achalasia. The definition of borderline IRP in this context ranges from 10 to 15 mm Hg with the Given Imaging system.

Distal Esophageal Spasm

Premature contractions, defined as having a DL less than 4.5 seconds, have been shown to be more specific than rapid contractions (defined as a CFV >9 cm/s) for the diagnosis of distal esophageal spasm.[18] The Working Group concluded that rapid contractions were so nonspecific that they should not be considered a significant abnormality. As a result it is now proposed that distal esophageal spasm be defined by the occurrence of greater than or equal to 20% premature contractions in a context of normal EGJ relaxation.

Jackhammer Esophagus

The definition of hypercontractile esophagus (nicknamed jackhammer esophagus) was based on the occurrence of at least 1 swallow with a DCI greater than 8000 mm Hg·s·cm in the 2012 Chicago Classification.[15] However, it has become apparent that this disorder is heterogeneous and might occur in the context of other esophageal abnormalities, such as EGJ outflow obstruction, gastroesophageal reflux

Table 5
Esophageal motility diagnoses and criteria proposed for the Chicago Classification v3.0

Disorders with EGJ outflow obstruction	Criteria
Type I achalasia (classic achalasia)	Increased median IRP (>15 mm Hg[a]), 100% failed peristalsis (DCI <100 mm Hg) Premature contractions with DCI values <450 mm Hg·s·cm meet criteria for failed peristalsis
Type II achalasia (with esophageal compression)	Increased median IRP (>15 mm Hg[a]), 100% failed peristalsis, panesophageal pressurization with ≥20% of swallows Contractions may be masked by esophageal pressurization and DCI should not be calculated
Type III achalasia (spastic achalasia)	Increased median IRP (>15 mm Hg[a]), no normal peristalsis, premature (spastic) contractions with DCI >450 mm Hg·s·cm with ≥20% of swallows May be mixed with panesophageal pressurization
EGJ outflow obstruction	Increased median IRP (>15 mm Hg[a]), sufficient evidence of peristalsis such that criteria for types I-III achalasia not met[b]
Major disorders of peristalsis	Not encountered in normal subjects
Aperistalsis	Normal median IRP, 100% failed peristalsis Should consider achalasia with borderline IRP values when there is evidence of esophageal pressurization Premature contractions with DCI values <450 mm Hg·s·cm meet criteria for failed peristalsis
Distal esophageal spasm	Normal median IRP, ≥20% premature contractions with DCI >450 mm Hg·s·cm[a]. Some normal peristalsis may be present
Hypercontractile esophagus (jackhammer)	At least 2 swallows with DCI >8000 mm Hg·s·cm[a,c] Hypercontractility may be localized to the LES and may be missed using DCI criteria
Minor disorders of peristalsis	Characterized by vigor, pattern, and MRS response
IEM	>50% ineffective swallows Ineffective swallows can be failed or weak Multiple repetitive swallow assessment may be helpful in determining peristaltic reserve
Fragmented peristalsis	>50% fragmented contractions not meeting IEM criteria
Normal esophageal motility	Not fulfilling any of the classifications listed earlier

Abbreviations: IEM, ineffective esophageal motility; MRS, multiple rapid swallowing.

[a] Cutoff value depends on the manometric hardware; this is the cutoff for the Given system.

[b] Potential causes: early achalasia, mechanical obstruction, esophageal wall stiffness, or manifestation of hiatal hernia, in which case it can be subtyped to CD or LES.

[c] Hypercontractile esophagus can be a manifestation of outflow obstruction, as shown by instances in which it occurs in association with an IRP greater than the upper limit of normal.

disease (GERD), or eosinophilic esophagitis. Furthermore, with one Working Group member's observation of an 8000 mm Hg·s·cm occurring in a control subject, the threshold of 1 swallow meeting that criterion was deemed insufficient and of uncertain relevance. Hence, the international HRM Working Group proposed to define jackhammer esophagus as the occurrence of greater than or equal to 20% of swallows with a DCI greater than 8000 mm Hg·s·cm. Another caveat that has come to light is that hypercontractility extended to the LES might be missed using strict DCI criteria. Hence, in some instances (such as that shown in **Fig. 6**), expanding the DCI measurement to include the EGJ may be warranted.

MINOR MOTILITY DISORDERS

The clinical significance of minor motility disorders continues to be debated. It was the strong feeling of the Working Group that overly classifying these was counterproductive because it distracted attention from the importance of identifying the major disorders. Hence, in order to improve this situation, it has been proposed to define minor motility disorders based on the contractile vigor, contractile pattern, and the response to multiple rapid swallows in the Chicago Classification v3.0.

Peristaltic Abnormalities as Defined in the 2012 Chicago Classification

The 2012 Chicago Classification listed 5 peristaltic abnormalities.

- Weak peristalsis with large peristaltic defects was defined by a normal IRP and greater than 20% of swallows with large breaks in the 20 mm Hg isobaric contour (>5 cm in length).
- Weak peristalsis with small peristaltic defects corresponded with normal IRP and greater than 30% of swallows with small breaks in the 20 mm Hg isobaric contour (2–5 cm in length).
- Frequent failed peristalsis was defined by greater than 30% but less than 100% of swallows with failed peristalsis.

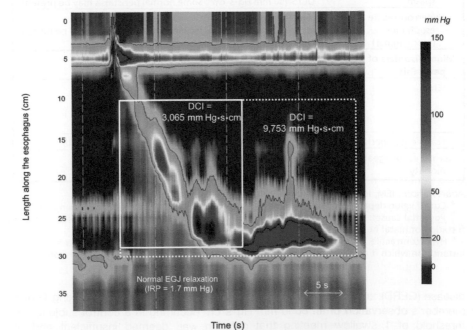

Fig. 6. Normal esophageal contraction followed by a prominent contraction of the LES. Including the EGJ in the DCI measurement (*white dashed box*) may result in the diagnosis of hypercontractility.

- Rapid contractions with normal latency corresponded with rapid contractions (CFV >9 cm/s and DL >4.5 s) with 20% of swallows.
- Hypertensive peristalsis was defined as a mean DCI greater than 5000 mm Hg·s·cm, but not meeting criteria for hypercontractile esophagus.

Limitations of the 2012 Chicago Classification

As alluded to earlier, the 2012 Chicago Classification for peristaltic abnormalities encountered significant dissatisfaction in the clinical community because of its complexity and because of the unclear relevance of the subtypes. For example, small peristaltic defects are common in healthy controls; Kumar and colleagues[22] observed that breaks reaching or exceeding 20% of the esophageal length in greater than or equal to 30% of test swallows was encountered in 27% of control subjects. The relevance of rapid contractions is also debated and unclear. Among 67 patients with at least 20% of rapid contractions with normal latency, Pandolfino and colleagues[18] showed that this abnormality was associated with EGJ outflow obstruction (n = 7, 11%), weak peristalsis (n = 41, 61%), hypertensive peristalsis (n = 5, 7%), and even normal peristalsis (n = 14, 21%). A substantial number of controls might also show rapid contractions. In addition, the relevance of hypertensive peristalsis is not widely accepted. Its definition, based on a mean DCI among 10 swallows being greater than 5000 mm Hg·s·cm, was inconsistent with the general scheme of the Chicago Classification that is otherwise based on the individual scoring of swallows. Furthermore, this value has significant overlap with control subjects.

Minor Motility Disorders Proposed for Chicago Classification v3.0

Given the limitations just described, the Working Group has proposed major simplifications to the definitions of minor motility disorders. Thus, all peristaltic abnormalities defined in the 2012 Chicago Classification have been abandoned. In their place, Chicago Classification v3.0 adopts the terminology ineffective esophageal motility (IEM), popularized in conventional manometric diagnoses, and fragmented peristalsis.

Ineffective Esophageal Motility

The unifying feature of swallows contributing to the diagnosis of IEM is poor bolus transit in the distal esophagus. Using conventional manometry, IEM was defined by 50% or more ineffective esophageal swallows, which were in turn defined as esophageal contractions with amplitudes less than 30 mm Hg at pressure sensors positioned 3 or 8 cm above the LES.[23] Correlating conventional line tracing analysis and Clouse plots analysis, Xiao and colleagues[24] showed that ineffective swallows (IES) on conventional line tracing potentially corresponded with a mixture of intact contractions (ie, a contraction without a break in the 20 mm Hg isobaric contour), weak contractions with small or large breaks, and failed contractions on Clouse plots. However, shifting to the criterion of a DCI less than 450 mm Hg·s·cm was optimal in predicting IES (positive percent agreement 83% and negative percent agreement 90% in a validation sample of 100 patients). Thus, it has been proposed to define ineffective swallows on Clouse plots by having a DCI less than 450 mm Hg·s·cm with more than 50% ineffective swallows constituting IEM. No distinction need be made between failed swallows and weak swallows.

Another recent development relevant to the diagnosis of IEM is that multiple rapid swallowing (MRS) has been proposed as a test to evaluate peristaltic reserve. MRS consists of administering five 2-mL water swallows separated by intervals of 2 to 3 seconds; too brief a period to allow significant peristaltic progression. MRS results in profound inhibition of the esophageal body and LES and is normally followed by an esophageal contraction of increased amplitude. Using conventional manometry, half of patients with IEM normalized esophageal contraction amplitude after MRS,[25] a phenomenon referred to as peristaltic reserve. Applying this concept to HRM, the DCI of the contraction that followed MRS was compared with the average DCI of the 10 test 5-mL water swallows in controls and in a cohort of patients with GERD before fundoplication.[26] The DCI ratio (DCI after MRS/average DCI of the 10 swallows) was greater than 1 in 78% of controls, 64% of patients without dysphagia after fundoplication, 44% of patients with early dysphagia after fundoplication, and 11% of patients with late dysphagia after fundoplication (P<.02). Further, a DCI ratio greater than 0.85 had a sensitivity of 67% and a specificity of 64% in segregating patients with late postoperative dysphagia from those with no postoperative dysphagia. Thus, the DCI ratio might reflect the peristaltic reserve and help predict the occurrence of postoperative dysphagia after antireflux surgery. The international HRM Working Group acknowledged the utility of MRS in patients with IEM to evaluate the peristaltic reserve, but it is not yet uncertain how it will be worked into the classification.

Fragmented Peristalsis

Even though breaks in the 20 mm Hg isobaric contours are frequently encountered in control subjects and patients, large breaks (>5 cm) might be clinically relevant. Large breaks are significantly more common in patients with dysphagia than in controls (14% vs 4%; P = .02).[27] Porter and colleagues showed that the proportion of failed or fragmented contractions was greater in patients with GERD than in controls (61.9% vs 33.3%; P≤.08). Because of the potential clinical relevance of large breaks, the Working Group has proposed to define fragmented peristalsis as greater than or equal to 50% fragmented contractions, with the added stipulation of not meeting IEM criteria.[28]

Normal Esophageal Motility

In addition, normal esophageal motility is considered if criteria for the motility disorders discussed earlier are not fulfilled.

WHAT IS IN THE FUTURE?

The Chicago Classification is an evolving process. Version 3.0 takes into account interval publications since 2012 and the worldwide clinical experience of experts. Definitions of esophageal dysmotility are simplified to facilitate their use in daily clinical practice. As with earlier iterations, these changes are intended to segregate clinically relevant disorders from statistically abnormal motility. In the future, additional findings will likely be incorporated that further improve accuracy and utility. The use of combined impedance HRM might be helpful to assess pharyngeal motility and UES function[29] and may also complement the analysis of esophageal function.[30,31] Performing HRM in alternative conditions such as upright posture[9,11] may also be considered because this may improve diagnostic yield. Swallow challenges introduced into the clinical study, such as free drinking[32] or a test meal,[33] to trigger motility abnormalities may similarly prove to be clinically relevant.

ACKNOWLEDGMENTS

This is a preliminary report of the transactions leading to and during the HRM Working Group meeting on HRM that transpired in Chicago on May 6 to 7, 2014. It represents a summary of the meeting as agreed on by the authors, but is still preliminary in that it has not yet gained the approval of the broader group. The international high resolution manometry working group is composed as follows,

Core members: Peter J Kahrilas*, Albert J Bredenoord, Mark Fox, C Prakash Gyawali, John E Pandolfino, Sabine Roman, AJPM Smout.

Working Group Members: Shobna Bhatia, Guy Boeckxstaens, Serhat Bor, DO Castell, Minhu Chen, Daniel Cisternas, Jeffrey L Conklin, Ian J Cook, Kerry Dunbar, Geoffrey Hebbard, Ikuo Hirano, Richard H Holloway, Phil Katz, David Katzka, Meiyun Ke, Jutta Keller, Anthony Lembo, Ravinder K Mittal, Taher Omari, Jeff Peters, Joel Richter, Nathalie Rommel, Renato Salvador, Edoardo Savarino, Felice Schnoll-Sussman, Werner Schwizer, Daniel Sifrim, Stuart Spechler, Rami Sweis, Jan Tack, Radu Tutuian, Miguel Valdovinos, Marcelo F Vela, Yinglian Xiao, Frank Zerbib.

REFERENCES

1. Soudagar AS, Sayuk GS, Gyawali CP. Learners favour high resolution oesophageal manometry with better diagnostic accuracy over conventional line tracings. Gut 2012;61(6):798–803.
2. Pandolfino JE, Fox MR, Bredenoord AJ, et al. High-resolution manometry in clinical practice: utilizing pressure topography to classify oesophageal motility abnormalities. Neurogastroenterol Motil 2009;21(8):796–806.
3. Bredenoord AJ, Fox M, Kahrilas PJ, et al. Chicago classification criteria of esophageal motility disorders defined in high resolution esophageal pressure topography (EPT). Neurogastroenterol Motil 2012;24(Suppl 1):57–65.
4. Bogte A, Bredenoord AJ, Oors J, et al. Normal values for esophageal high-resolution manometry. Neurogastroenterol Motil 2013;25(9):762.e579.
5. Ghosh SK, Pandolfino JE, Rice J, et al. Impaired deglutitive EGJ relaxation in clinical esophageal manometry: a quantitative analysis of 400 patients and 75 controls. Am J Physiol Gastrointest Liver Physiol 2007;293(4):G878–85.
6. Ghosh SK, Pandolfino JE, Zhang Q, et al. Quantifying esophageal peristalsis with high-resolution manometry: a study of 75 asymptomatic volunteers. Am J Physiol Gastrointest Liver Physiol 2006;290(5):G988–97.
7. Kessing BF, Weijenborg PW, Smout AJ, et al. Water-perfused esophageal high-resolution manometry: normal values and validation. Am J Physiol Gastrointest Liver Physiol 2014;306(6):G491–5.
8. Niebisch S, Wilshire CL, Peters JH. Systematic analysis of esophageal pressure topography in high-resolution manometry of 68 normal volunteers. Dis Esophagus 2013;26(7):651–60.
9. Sweis R, Anggiansah A, Wong T, et al. Normative values and inter-observer agreement for liquid and solid bolus swallows in upright and supine positions as assessed by esophageal high-resolution manometry. Neurogastroenterol Motil 2011;23(6):509.e198.
10. Weijenborg PW, Kessing BF, Smout AJ, et al. Normal values for solid-state esophageal high-resolution manometry in a European population; an overview of all current metrics. Neurogastroenterol Motil 2014;26(5):654–9.
11. Xiao Y, Read A, Nicodeme F, et al. The effect of a sitting vs supine posture on normative esophageal pressure topography metrics and Chicago classification diagnosis of esophageal motility disorders. Neurogastroenterol Motil 2012; 24(10):e509–16.

---

* Chairperson

12. Pandolfino JE, Kim H, Ghosh SK, et al. High-resolution manometry of the EGJ: an analysis of crural diaphragm function in GERD. Am J Gastroenterol 2007;102(5): 1056–63.
13. Bredenoord AJ, Weusten BL, Timmer R, et al. Intermittent spatial separation of diaphragm and lower esophageal sphincter favors acidic and weakly acidic reflux. Gastroenterology 2006;130(2):334–40.
14. Xiao Y, Kahrilas PJ, Nicodeme F, et al. Lack of correlation between HRM metrics and symptoms during the manometric protocol. Am J Gastroenterol 2014;109(4): 521–6.
15. Roman S, Pandolfino JE, Chen J, et al. Phenotypes and clinical context of hypercontractility in high resolution pressure topography (EPT). Am J Gastroenterol 2012;107(1):37–45.
16. Pandolfino JE, Leslie E, Luger D, et al. The contractile deceleration point: an important physiologic landmark on oesophageal pressure topography. Neurogastroenterol Motil 2010;22(4):395–400.
17. Lin Z, Pandolfino JE, Xiao Y, et al. Localizing the contractile deceleration point (CDP) in patients with abnormal esophageal pressure topography. Neurogastroenterol Motil 2012;24(10):972–5.
18. Pandolfino JE, Roman S, Carlson D, et al. Distal esophageal spasm in high-resolution esophageal pressure topography: defining clinical phenotypes. Gastroenterology 2011;141(2):469–75.
19. Pandolfino JE, Kwiatek MA, Nealis T, et al. Achalasia: a new clinically relevant classification by high-resolution manometry. Gastroenterology 2008;135(5): 1526–33.
20. Lin Z, Kahrilas PJ, Roman S, et al. Refining the criterion for an abnormal Integrated Relaxation Pressure in esophageal pressure topography based on the pattern of esophageal contractility using a classification and regression tree model. Neurogastroenterol Motil 2012;24(8):e356–63.
21. Roman S, Kahrilas PJ, Mion F, et al. Partial recovery of peristalsis after myotomy for achalasia: more the rule than the exception. JAMA Surg 2013;148(2): 157–64.
22. Kumar N, Porter RF, Chanin JM, et al. Analysis of intersegmental trough and proximal latency of smooth muscle contraction using high-resolution esophageal manometry. J Clin Gastroenterol 2012;46(5):375–81.
23. Blonski W, Vela M, Safder A, et al. Revised criterion for diagnosis of ineffective esophageal motility is associated with more frequent dysphagia and greater bolus transit abnormalities. Am J Gastroenterol 2008;103(3):699–704.
24. Xiao Y, Kahrilas PJ, Kwasny MJ, et al. High-resolution manometry correlates of ineffective esophageal motility. Am J Gastroenterol 2012;107(11):1647–54.
25. Fornari F, Bravi I, Penagini R, et al. Multiple rapid swallowing: a complementary test during standard oesophageal manometry. Neurogastroenterol Motil 2009; 21(7):718.e41.
26. Shaker A, Stoikes N, Drapekin J, et al. Multiple rapid swallow responses during esophageal high-resolution manometry reflect esophageal body peristaltic reserve. Am J Gastroenterol 2013;108(11):1706–12.
27. Roman S, Lin Z, Kwiatek MA, et al. Weak peristalsis in esophageal pressure topography: classification and association with dysphagia. Am J Gastroenterol 2011;106(2):349–56.
28. Porter RF, Kumar N, Drapekin JE, et al. Fragmented esophageal smooth muscle contraction segments on high resolution manometry: a marker of esophageal hypomotility. Neurogastroenterol Motil 2012;24:763–e353.

29. Omari TI, Dejaeger E, van Beckevoort D, et al. A method to objectively assess swallow function in adults with suspected aspiration. Gastroenterology 2011; 140(5):1454–63.
30. Lin Z, Imam H, Nicodeme F, et al. Flow time through esophagogastric junction derived during high-resolution impedance-manometry studies: a novel parameter for assessing esophageal bolus transit. Am J Physiol Gastrointest Liver Physiol 2014. [Epub ahead of print].
31. Rommel N, Van Oudenhove L, Tack J, et al. Automated impedance manometry analysis as a method to assess esophageal function. Neurogastroenterol Motil 2014;26(5):636–45.
32. Daum C, Sweis R, Kaufman E, et al. Failure to respond to physiologic challenge characterizes esophageal motility in erosive gastro-esophageal reflux disease. Neurogastroenterol Motil 2011;23(6):517.e200.
33. Sweis R, Anggiansah A, Wong T, et al. Assessment of esophageal dysfunction and symptoms during and after a standardized test meal: development and clinical validation of a new methodology utilizing high-resolution manometry. Neurogastroenterol Motil 2014;26(2):215–28.

The Role of Barium Esophagography in an Endoscopy World

David A. Katzka, MD

KEYWORDS

- Esophagography • Esophagram • Radiology

KEY POINTS

- Barium radiography is a powerful tool in its ability to combine critical analysis of esophageal motility, relative replication of patient physiologic swallowing function, good anatomic definition and the ability to correlate potential symptoms with findings on imaging.
- Use of barium in a video swallow study remains the best test to diagnose and often treat disorders of oropharyngeal dysfunction.
- Barium radiography is an important research role in elucidating normal function of the oropharynx, particularly when used with other modalities such as high-resolution manometry and impedance.

INTRODUCTION

Barium esophagography is not pretty. It does not offer the imaginative cross-sectional images and 3-dimensional reconstructions of newer radiologic software. It does not generate the excitement and control of holding an endoscopic instrument coupled with new light-filtering devices and greater diagnostic and therapeutic potential. It also involves consuming a rather unpleasant fluid. On the other hand, in the skills of a seasoned gastrointestinal radiologist, there is no esophageal test that better combines critical analysis of esophageal motility, relative replication of patient physiologic swallowing function, good anatomic definition, and ability to correlate potential symptoms with findings on imaging.

TERMINOLOGY

In discussing the role of barium studies as a complement to endoscopy in the diagnosis of esophageal disorders, we must first define the terms used to characterize

Disclosure: The authors have nothing to disclose.
Division of Gastroenterology and Hepatology, Mayo Clinic, 200 First Avenue Southwest, Rochester, MN 55905, USA
E-mail address: Katzka.david@mayo.edu

Gastrointest Endoscopy Clin N Am 24 (2014) 563–580
http://dx.doi.org/10.1016/j.giec.2014.06.004
1052-5157/14/$ – see front matter © 2014 Elsevier Inc. All rights reserved.

the specific types of studies that can be ordered. Indeed, this may be one of the most misunderstood aspects of barium esophagography in which the catchall phrase, "an UGI" is commonly used to refer to several distinct methods of measuring esophageal function and anatomy. One cannot reinforce enough the need to understand the methods of these examinations so that the physician may obtain the proper and needed information to diagnose the individual patient's esophageal disorder.

Video Swallow Study

This study has many alternative names, which include video fluoroscopic swallowing study, video fluoroscopic swallowing evaluation, or a modified barium swallow. In this study, the patient is asked to swallow various types of substances, such as thin and thick barium and cookies or crackers that can be seen by fluoroscopy to evaluate his or her ability to swallow. It is commonly performed with a speech and swallowing therapist who lends not only expertise to performance and interpretation of the study, but may also initiate and plan therapeutic maneuvers based on this study. This study focuses exclusively on the oropharynx and proximal esophagus.

Esophagram

With the use of thin barium, this study is used to visualize the anatomic structural and motility aspects of the esophagus. It can be performed as either a single and/or double contrast study. With the exception of specific circumstances (eg, single contrast only such as evaluation of a tracheoesophageal fistula or Schatzki ring), most esophagrams are performed with both these techniques starting with single contrast. This study focuses exclusively on the esophagus. A cine esophagram refers to video recording of the esophagram rather than using only still images.

PERFORMANCE OF THE EXAMINATION

Performance of barium radiography involves 2 key principles: The use of both single and double contrast techniques and rotation of the patient into multiple positions to best visualize structures.[1] Double contrast, using an effervescent agent after barium, is performed first, followed by a single contrast study. The former method is helpful for mucosal detail, whereas the latter is helpful in measuring esophageal diameter both generally and in the presence of strictured areas. Multiple positions are used, such as upright or prone, anteroposterior, and oblique. Multiple swallows of barium contrast are given in each of these positions. All swallows are observed through fluoroscopy, presumably from the initial phases of swallow to entry into the stomach. Indeed, it is the skill of the radiologist in using these methods and views to achieve optimal visualization of the esophagus and its disorders.

THEORETIC ADVANTAGES OF RADIOGRAPHY COMPARED WITH ENDOSCOPY

By administration of oral contrast and fluoroscopic imaging, the esophagram offers several advantages over endoscopy. The first advantage is that an assessment of esophageal motility and function can be made.[2] Correlation of esophageal radiography to esophageal manometry is generally excellent for a number of functions. For example, the mechanical correlate of peristalsis is of a stripping wave that milks the esophagus clean from its proximal to distal end. The velocity of the stripping wave corresponds closely with that of the manometrically recorded contractile pattern. More specifically, the upstroke of the pressure wave corresponds with the point of the inverted "V" (the leading edge of the column of barium as seen fluoroscopically). The efficacy of distal esophageal emptying is closely related to peristaltic amplitude, such that emptying becomes progressively impaired with peristaltic amplitudes of 30 mm Hg[2] or less. Further measures of esophageal emptying may include the height of the barium column and the time it takes for the esophagus to empty a standard quantity of swallowed barium.[3] This value can be particularly helpful in monitoring disorders that cause functional or mechanical esophageal obstruction. This threshold amplitude was initially determined from simultaneous videofluoroscopic and manometric recordings of a relatively small number of subjects Visualization of swallowing radiographically also provides information on both longitudinal and circular muscle shortening. Furthermore, when evaluating whether there is symptom dependence on bolus type, studies using simultaneous radiography and manometry have demonstrated that more a more viscous bolus increases contraction duration, but not amplitude, corresponding with slower transit through the esophagus. It is also important to note that, as in manometry, normal volunteers may not have complete bolus transit on all swallows and remain asymptomatic. These are some of the finer points of evaluating esophageal motility by barium administration.

Barium administration also gives a detailed view of lower esophageal sphincter (LES) opening, closing, and flow through the gastroesophageal junction.[4,5] In contrast with manometry, which may measure LES relaxation through pressure measurement, radiography gives a more accurate measure of LES opening. This is an important distinguishing point, because LES relaxation relates to neuropeptide mediated inhibition of LES contraction, whereas sphincter opening depends on additional factors, such as the strength of antegrade peristaltic force as seen on imaging. A reasonable estimate of LES tone is also possible, either by measuring stasis of contrast proximal to an LES that fails to open adequately, or, in contrast, a freely open or "patulous" sphincter, which allows free retrograde flow of barium, particularly in the recumbent position or when associated with hiatal hernia.[6] Although the relationship of reflux measured on pH/impedance studies to contrast radiography is often tenuous, when marked reflux on barium to the thoracic inlet occurs, studies have shown there is good correlation with marked recumbent reflux on pH studies.

A second advantage of barium radiography is the ability to give a more accurate assessment of esophageal luminal diameter. Studies using endoscopy to assess lumen size have been disappointing demonstrating underestimation or overestimation in a large number of patients. In contrast, radiographic images allow direct measurement of esophageal diameter. This allows for more accurate determination of the length, location, and number of dilated and/or narrowed areas of the esophagus. Furthermore, measurement of minimal and maximal luminal diameters is possible in an individual patient, giving a rough measure of wall distensibility and compliance.

A third advantage of radiography is the ability to change the texture and size of the swallowed bolus to fit the clinical information desired. Stated another way, by administration of a liquid (barium), semisolid (barium paste), or a solid (barium tablet or cookie) to a patient with dysphagia, one has the ability to corroborate a symptom referable to a specific type of bolus with an objective finding. Furthermore, on delayed transit of a radiographically visible bolus, one can ask the patient if and where the sensation of dysphagia occurred. Similarly, if expression of dysphagia occurs without obvious delay in esophageal transit, radiography may establish a sensory rather than obstructive etiology as a cause of symptoms.

A fourth advantage of barium esophagography is to give further insight into lesions that result in esophageal compression. Although endoscopy may visualize impingement of the esophageal lumen from a structure under normal overlying mucosa, its ability to determine precise etiology and location is limited. Barium imaging allows for better delineation of size as well as differentiation of intramural or extrinsic processes; the effect of the abnormality on the wall and not just the mucosa of the esophagus is more clearly seen. Furthermore, imaging of surrounding structures that can impinge on the esophagus, such as the cervical spine or heart, can be seen well during esophagography, giving further information on the cause of compression.

A fifth advantage of esophagography is that it may help to plan and make safer the ultimate need for endoscopy. For example, in patients in whom achalasia has already been diagnosed by esophagography, only 1 endoscopy is needed at which time therapeutic maneuvers such as injection of botulinum toxin or pneumatic dilation may be performed. Endoscopic ultrasonography may also be scheduled simultaneously for better evaluation of submucosal lesions or the need to rule out secondary causes of achalasia. For multiple or complex strictures, advanced planning such as need for fluoroscopy, a rendezvous procedure or anesthesia assistance may be implemented. For proximal unexpected lesions such as a Zenker diverticulum, a cervical web or a tight proximal stricture from lichen planus or eosinophilic esophagitis (EoE), endoscopic perforation may be better avoided.

THE USE OF BARIUM ESOPHAGOGRAPHY IN SPECIFIC ESOPHAGEAL DISORDERS
Oropharyngeal Dysfunction

A strong advantage of a barium study when compared with endoscopy is the ability to visualize oropharyngeal function. Whereas endoscopy gives strictly an anatomic assessment of this area, barium is more advantageous from a clinical point of view, where the majority of disorders that affect swallowing in this area result from dysmotility of neuromuscular origin. Furthermore, video esophagography is accurate in isolating the specific stages of swallowing and the muscle groups assigned to these phases, including tongue motion and other oral aspects of swallowing. As a result, there is a marked potential to determine a precise pathophysiology and, consequently, an etiology in patients with oropharyngeal dysphagia unlikely with endoscopy in the absence of structural deformity.[7] Specifically, one can isolate disorders of asymmetric weakness or nonuniform weakness reflecting selective neuropathic dysfunction as opposed to global dysfunction as a result of diffuse myopathy or neuropathy. There are also specific characteristics on video swallow that might further give insight into the disease process. This might include finding of a cricopharyngeal bar more commonly associated with diseases, such as myopathies/myositis (particularly inclusion body myositis), postpolio syndrome, brainstem stroke, and oculopharyngeal dystrophy.

With dysfunction of the oropharyngeal musculature, this study also accurately assesses the patient's ability to eat. This assessment depends generally on the 2 main functions described with this study: Adequate transport of barium bolus from mouth to esophagus and avoidance of aspiration. The latter is particularly important where a study has shown that aspiration on modified barium swallow is a strong predictor of subsequent clinical.[8] Furthermore, the density and texture of the swallowed bolus may be varied to test a variety of eating conditions. For example, during a video swallow, both thin and thick barium and solids such as cookies or tablets are given, because the oropharynx may handle these substances differently. This may be of clinical importance in structuring a diet for a patient where free aspiration of thin liquids may occur, but more successful swallowing of denser substances is seen. In addition to alteration of diet, a video swallow, when performed in the presence of a speech and swallowing therapist, also allows for the teaching of therapeutic maneuvers and exercises for both short- and long-term improvement of swallowing function. Similarly, particularly when performed with an expert radiologist and/or speech and swallow therapist, this type of radiography encourages valuable exchange of compatible but different information on swallowing ability, leading to a more comprehensive approach to a patient's swallowing needs. Needless to say, this test contributes important information that could not be achieved with endoscopic imaging alone.

Zenker Diverticulum

A Zenker diverticulum (**Fig. 1**) is a posterior pharyngoesophageal pouch that forms through pulsion forces in an area of relative hypopharyngeal wall weakness between the oblique fibers of the inferior pharyngeal constrictor and the horizontal fibers of the cricopharyngeus muscles.[9] As in any diverticulum, the complete anatomy of the outpouching is best seen on a barium study, where full filling of the diverticulum by contrast occurs. Furthermore, one is not deterred by fear of perforation or inability to transverse the neck of the diverticulum, as may occur with endoscopy. Visualization of this area of diverticulum formation is also easier with barium, because the space between the cricopharyngeus and inferior pharyngeal constrictor is poorly tolerated during routine endoscopy unless deep sedation is used.

A barium study performed for evaluation of Zenker diverticulum is also valuable in planning surgery. For example, factors such as the size and location of the diverticulum may determine the use of an endoscopic, transoral rigid, or open approach to repair. The contrast study also better visualizes the cricopharyngeus muscle, which is commonly prominent on imaging owing to fibrosis and poor compliance, thus leading to increased pharyngeal pressures and development of the diverticulum. Indeed, intubation of the esophagus past this "bar" may be difficult and, conversely, may not be appreciated as diseased. It is also important to note that not all hypopharyngeal diverticula are Zenker diverticula; for example, a Killian-Jamieson diverticulum[10] may have a similar appearance endoscopically but require a different operative approach when more easily diagnosed by contrast esophagography.

Gastroesophageal Reflux Disease

One of the more controversial areas in the diagnosis of gastroesophageal reflux disease (GERD) is the meaning of reflux of barium in relation to clinically important

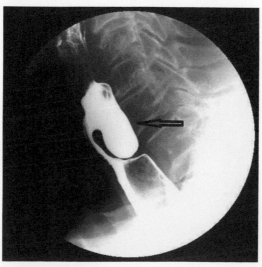

Fig. 1. Zenker diverticulum (*arrow*).

gastroesophageal reflux (**Fig. 2**). For many years, radiologists used maneuvers to provoke reflux of barium, including increasing abdominal pressure by a binder or by water siphon test. In the water siphon test, patients are asked to swallow 60 mL of water and then are changed in position during fluoroscopy to provoke reflux of barium into the esophagus. When typical reflux symptoms are used as a gold standard, the water siphon test can be sensitive and specific, even when compared with ambulatory pH monitoring.[11] With regard to free reflux of barium seen during an UGI series, others have also shown good correlation with pathologic reflux seen during ambulatory pH monitoring.[12] This is in contrast with endoscopy where clear indications of GERD such as erosive esophagitis or stricture formation are found in only a minority of patients. Unfortunately, the potential excellent sensitivity of barium radiography for diagnosing GERD is accompanied by low specificity. Many factors explain the low specificity, such as the lack of physiologic correlation of barium with food or the provoked maneuvers to actual pathophysiology. Furthermore, there is no gold standard for how much and to what proximal extent of barium reflux occurring constitutes an accurate diagnosis of GERD. As a result, reflux of barium as a means of diagnosing GERD is considered limited except with perhaps free reflux of barium to high proximal levels, such as the thoracic inlet, where there is good correlation to pathologic pH monitoring results in some.[12]

A barium study may also be useful in diagnosing GERD in terms of structural abnormalities identified. For example, identification of a distal esophageal stricture in a middle-aged man with years of heartburn provides excellent evidence for severe GERD. Unfortunately, as in endoscopic signs of esophageal injury from GERD, this is found in a minority of patients. Identification of a large sliding hiatal hernia may also be helpful. Although finding a hernia per se does not define the presence of GERD, the association of a hernia of large size with reflux can be important in substantiating symptoms. Similar, other radiographic signs such as a widely patent gastroesophageal junction may be supportive of GERD but by no means have been studied well enough to make it a pathognomonic sign of GERD. The other important aspect of measuring hernia size by radiography is in measuring esophageal length

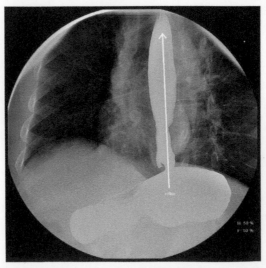

Fig. 2. Radiographic demonstration of reflux of barium (*arrow*) into the esophagus.

above the hernia. High degrees of esophageal shortening commonly associated with hiatal hernia and chronic severe GERD may dictate the need for an esophageal lengthening procedure with operative therapy.

One of the most helpful aspects of barium radiology, in contrast with endoscopy, is differentiating a sliding from a paraesophageal hernia. Although symptomatically these hernias may differ in presentation, often the larger hernias are mixed with symptoms of both reflux from the sliding component and obstruction and ischemia from the paraesophageal portion in individual patients. Identification of a paraesophageal hernia is crucial given the threat of incarceration accompanied by high morbidity and mortality. Radiography gives a more accurate view of these hernias compared with endoscopy, given the ability to better visualize the relationship of the diaphragm to the hernia, the location of the gastroesophageal junction relative to the hernia, and if paraesophageal, the type of hernia present. This also applies to other types of diaphragmatic hernias such as Bochdalek and Morgagni.

Finally, barium esophagography is more accurate than endoscopy in characterizing the flaccid, dilated, patulous esophagus commonly found in patients with scleroderma. Recognition of this disease as a cause of refractory reflux symptoms and/or esophagitis is essential, because fundoplication is generally contraindicated in these patients and high-dose proton pump inhibitor therapy is needed.

Schatzki Ring

A Schatzki ring is a circumferential, protruding ring of mucosa at the squamocolumnar junction that compromises luminal size and causes solid food and pill dysphagia based largely on the side of the residual esophageal diameter (**Fig. 3**). It is putatively a reflux-induced lesion, but clear data supporting this theory is lacking. In patients where there is obvious impingement of the ring on esophageal diameter, endoscopically readily diagnoses this lesion. In many patients, however, appearance of the ring may be subtle and only appreciated with maximal distention of the gastroesophageal junction endoscopically, a maneuver that is not always accomplished during the procedure. As a result, barium esophagography, particularly when

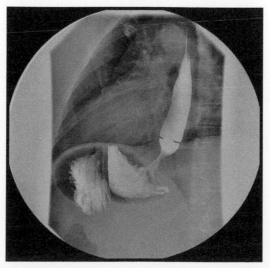

Fig. 3. Schatzki ring.

performed in the prone position with single contrast technique, may be more accurate in detecting Schatzki rings than endoscopy.[13] In addition to the presence of the ring, esophagography may also identify the width of the ring. Indeed, some rings seem to be thicker (**Fig. 4**), suggesting a greater degree of fibrosis and esophageal wall involvement portending greater risk of perforation as opposed to rupturing mucosa alone. Indeed, some might term this a stricture rather than a ring, mandating chronic antireflux therapy, although there are no data to definitively support this recommendation.

Postfundoplication Syndromes

Postoperative and commonly persistent symptoms are commonly found after performance of a fundoplication. As a colleague of mine, Dr. Francis X. Nichols, states, undergoing fundoplication is "trading one set of symptoms for another." Similarly, the failure rate of fundoplication for control of heartburn can range up to 60% in long-term follow-up.[14] As a result, assessment is often needed to determine the efficacy of the fundoplication as reflected by its anatomic appearance. Several findings are commonly seen radiographically as potential complications of a fundoplication. The first is a tight fundoplication seen in evaluation for postoperative dysphagia. This remains somewhat controversial because there is no set diameter of the gastroesophageal junction below which dysphagia is likely. In fact, in some studies, the most reliable predictor of postfundoplication dysphagia is the presence of preoperative dysphagia. Other factors that have been shown to commonly predict postoperative dysphagia include ineffective esophageal motility, the degree of the wrap, and the type of fundoplication performed. In any case, short of taking down the fundoplication, many patients with dysphagia undergo endoscopic dilation of the wrap. Radiographically, without being too specific, one generally looks for a narrowed area through the fundoplication with a static, slowly draining column of barium above.

A rare scenario, which does lead to immediate, severe, and sustained postoperative dysphagia, is the development of achalasia secondary to the wrap. Barium

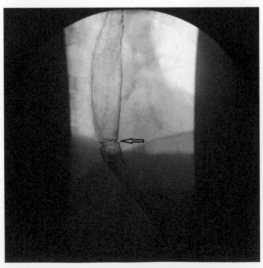

Fig. 4. Annular stricture with appearance of thick Schatzki ring (*arrow*).

esophagography demonstrates a tight and often bird beak area at the location of the fundoplication with a dilated esophagus above. The degree of dilation may be mild or moderate, but the esophagus remains straight, in contrast with chronic primary achalasia, which can commonly result in greater degrees of dilation and tortuosity. In this author's experience, these patients often need aggressive dilation, commonly with a pneumatic dilator, if not surgical revision.

Another common finding after fundoplication and well-visualized radiographically is herniation. This may be found early or late in the postoperative period. Indeed, a hernia may be seen decades after prior fundoplication, but the point of time in which it developed is unclear without radiographic follow-up. This herniation may take 2 forms. The first is recurrence of a preoperative sliding hiatal hernia. This is seen radiographically at a "slipped" fundoplication in which wrap can be seen surrounding the proximal stomach with proximal movement of the gastroesophageal junction into the chest **(Fig. 5)**. This is more common in patients with long-standing and severe reflux in which they have a shortened esophagus that cannot reliably withstand the stretch required to fashion the fundoplication below the diaphragm. At times, the hernia may be mild, however, despite a significant slippage of the wrap distally onto the stomach. The second type of herniation is paraesophageal, in which a part of the proximal stomach herniates alongside the wrap **(Fig. 6)**. These patients present, differently with more prandial and postprandial pain, in contrast with recurrent reflux after a slipped fundoplication. Both these herniations, however, commonly present with dysphagia. Sometimes large, complex, and combined hernias may occur after fundoplication.

Finally, a fistula develops rarely after fundoplication and is easily visualized with a barium study **(Fig. 7)**. These tend to occur after reoperations, particularly when multiple revision attempts are made. A fistula may course from the distal esophagus to the

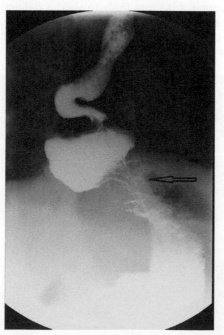

Fig. 5. Post-Nissen fundoplication herniation. *Arrow* denotes fundoplication.

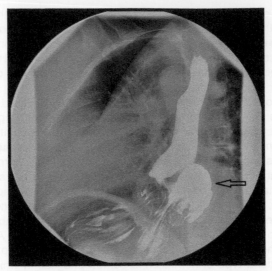

Fig. 6. Post-Nissen fundoplication with paraesophageal herniation (*arrow*).

proximal stomach bypassing the fundoplication or to the pleura or lung. This finding usually mandates treatment of an aggressive nature, sometimes leading to esophagectomy.

Achalasia

Barium esophagography holds a secure place in the diagnosis of achalasia. When compared with endoscopy, it is more likely to yield a definitive diagnosis given its greater sensitivity for esophageal dilation and the ability to measure LES opening. Indeed, studies have demonstrated that a normal esophageal endoscopic appearance is not uncommon in achalasia.[15] This is not surprising given the superior ability

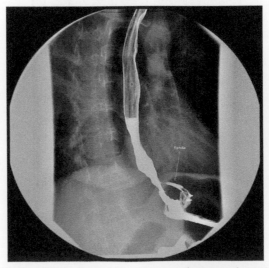

Fig. 7. Postfundoplication fistula (*arrow*) between esophagus and proximal stomach.

of radiography to measure esophageal diameter, assess esophageal motility, and visualize stasis of esophageal content. Although the LES may be characterized by a distinct "pop" upon traversing with the endoscope, the evident smooth narrowing on a contrast esophagram (bird beak) is far more convincing of the diagnosis. Radiography is also helpful in "staging" the disease. Although high-resolution esophageal manometry may provide some prognostic information based on the Chicago classification,[16] radiographic parameters, such as degree of dilation and sigmoidization (**Fig. 8**), are also important in prognosis and planning therapy. This is particularly true when weighing the therapeutic options of myotomy and esophagectomy for suspected end-stage disease. Part of this staging may also include the presence of an esophageal diverticulum. Appreciation of a diverticulum, better seen on radiography than endoscopy, is also important in determining therapy (**Fig. 9**). Specifically, the presence of an epiphrenic diverticulum is a relative contraindication to pneumatic dilation. The size of the diverticulum also influences the type of surgery (need for diverticulectomy) and the side of the esophagus on which the myotomy can be performed. Finally, barium esophagography to diagnose achalasia before endoscopy may allow for 1 less endoscopy by enabling planning of therapy during the endoscopy. For example, in patients with known achalasia by radiography, injection of botulinum toxin or pneumatic dilation may be performed during the initial endoscopy.

Barium esophagography also is important in assessing response to therapy through the "timed barium swallow."[3] In this test, while standing, patients ingest an amount of barium they can tolerate without regurgitation or aspiration (usually between 100 and 250 mL). Radiographs are taken at 1, 2, and 5 minutes after the last swallow of barium. The distance in centimeters from the distal esophagus (identified by the bird's beak appearance of the esophagogastric junction) to the top of a distinct barium column (barium height) as well as the maximal esophageal width were measured. Barium height is measured at 5 minutes to determine completeness of emptying. In this study, early relapse of symptoms was well defined by patients with abnormal emptying despite good symptomatic response initially. Further studies have also confirmed the predictive value of timed barium swallow postoperatively in

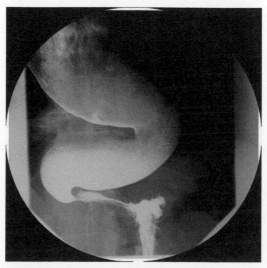

Fig. 8. Advanced stage achalasia with sigmoidization.

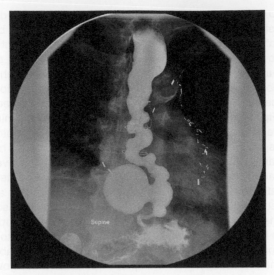

Fig. 9. Achalasia with epiphrenic diverticulum.

determining which patients are more likely to fail therapy and need subsequent intervention.[17]

STRICTURING DISEASES
EoE

EoE commonly manifests with esophageal strictures in the adult population. Indeed, 90% of adults with EoE present with dysphagia as their primary symptom. Endoscopically, rings and strictures may be seen in approximately 60% and 15% to 57% of EoE patients, respectively.[18–20] In these patients, barium studies have been shown to be far more sensitive in identifying esophageal strictures (**Fig. 10**). The techniques used

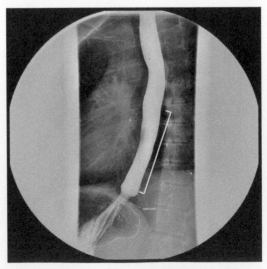

Fig. 10. Eosinophilic esophagitis with subtle long stricture (*arrow*).

to assess for strictures may include not only a direct visualization of the stricture but through a more subtle technique in which the minimum and maximal esophageal diameters are measured in response to barium ingestion. This gives a rough estimate of esophageal compliance or stiffness. In 1 study using this technique.[21] In these patients, barium studies have been shown to be far more sensitive in finding esophageal strictures with abnormalities detected in more than 50% of EoE patients.[21] Furthermore, these measurements were useful in detecting a favorable response to steroids. Finally, in my experience a well-performed barium study may detect the presence of subtle strictures, and is also accurate in assessing the details, such as diameter, length, and the superimposition of rings on strictures (**Fig. 11**) when compared with endoscopy in patients with EoE. This can be helpful in planning endoscopic therapy, such as the type of dilator to be used and where extra caution must be taken.

Lichen Planus

Lichen planus of the esophagus is another stricturing disease in which barium radiography is useful.[22] Although endoscopic recognition of characteristic mucosal findings, such as sloughing, whitish discoloration, and plaques, may not be appreciated on an esophagram, stricture is found in almost all patients with symptoms and may occur anywhere in the esophagus (**Fig. 12**). As a result, barium remains an important study in these patients. Furthermore, characterization of the stricture in these patients is essential in planning endoscopy given the risk of Koebnerization and paradoxic worsening of the stricture in overaggressive dilation or perhaps dilation in patients with active mucosal disease. Additionally, similar to patients with EoE, small caliber esophagus is not uncommon in lichen planus and best appreciated on radiography.

Caustic Injury

Similar to other stricturing diseases, barium esophagography is useful in more accurately determining the length and diameter of a caustic stricture.[23] This may be important when deciding on the method of dilation or stenting to be used. It is also important

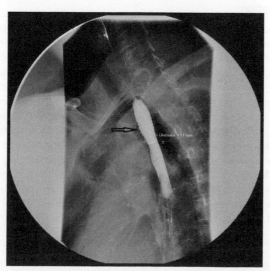

Fig. 11. Eosinophilic esophagitis with stricture and corrugated appearance (*arrow*).

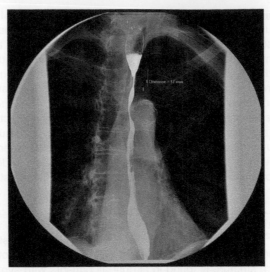

Fig. 12. Lichen planus with tight proximal esophageal stricture.

when considering operative options and staging the extent of disease when determining where an anastomosis may be formed. Similarly, a video swallow study is also essential in these patients; oropharyngeal function is commonly compromised in caustic ingestion. This is needed to assess risk of aspiration and implementation of swallowing maneuvers and exercises. It is also mandatory to prove that oropharyngeal function is normal in these patients before considering esophageal resection for severe caustic esophageal injury. Finally, in patients with acute severe caustic injury, a barium rather than endoscopic study is commonly used to assess the esophagus during the "latent" period (approximately 10–30 days after ingestion) where the chance of esophageal perforation with endoscopy is considerable owing to smoldering injury and remodeling.

Esophageal Perforation

The most common cause of esophageal perforation is iatrogenic, but may also result from many other causes including ingestion of a sharp or caustic foreign body (eg, fishbone, button battery), spontaneous rupture from vomiting and/or food impaction (Boorhaave syndrome), or trauma (eg, gunshot or stab wound). Diagnostic endoscopy is relatively contraindicated in these patients owing to fear of exacerbating the perforation. Esophagography, first with gastrograffin, and in the case of a confined leak, followed by barium, is a far more accurate and safer means of characterizing the size and extent of the perforation. This includes determination of whether the perforation is confined to the esophageal wall or periesophageal as opposed to free flow into the mediastinum or pleural cavity. Knowledge of these factors in planning therapy is essential; a confined perforation may be treated conservatively, whereas free perforation may require stenting and drainage or operative exploration and bypass. Subsequent esophageal imaging may also be useful to assess effective closure of the perforation by ongoing treatment, such as stent placement and with conservative management.

Esophageal Disorders Owing to Vascular Compression

Dysphagia may result from luminal compression by vascular structures adjacent to the esophagus. In older patients, the right atrium or a thoracic aortic aneurysm (dysphagia aortica) may compromise esophageal diameter and cause solid food dysphagia. Although extrinsic compression with pulsation may be appreciated on endoscopy, noninvasive and firm diagnosis of dysphagia aortica only occurs with radiographic imaging. Another vascular structure that may impinge on the esophagus and is not well appreciated on endoscopy is an aberrant right subclavian artery crossing over the esophagus, known as dysphagia lusoria. Although the clinical meaning of this abnormality is questioned and often viewed as an incidental abnormality in many patients, dysphagia may be associated with this congenital abnormality. Radiographically, a longitudinal smooth indentation is seen traversing the proximal esophagus in a diagonal fashion. Confirmation of the diagnosis can be made with cross sectional vascular imaging such as computed tomography or magnetic resonance imaging.

Miscellaneous Disorders

Nasogastric tube strictures are uncommon now owing to the use of these tubes for relatively short periods of time when compared with prior decades. The mechanism by which these strictures form in response to nasogastric tubes is unclear. Nevertheless, such strictures can be extensive, both in length and luminal compromise and are notably difficult to treat (**Fig. 13**). As in other diseases that result in a small caliber esophagus, barium esophagography gives more detailed information and is more helpful in planning endoscopic and/or surgical therapy than diagnostic endoscopy.

Although an esophageal diverticulum is most likely to occur in the hypopharyngeal or distal esophagus, other types of diverticula have been described and are better appreciated on barium esophagography. For example, intramural diverticulosis (**Fig. 14**) seems to be a nonspecific reaction associated with stricture formation. Strictures secondary to reflux, EoE, and idiopathic strictures have all been described with these intramural outpouchings.[24] These diverticula may represent dilated submucous glands, but there is also the anecdotal fear that the presence of these diverticula portend a higher chance of esophageal perforation with dilation. A single esophageal diverticulum may also form in the mid esophagus (**Fig. 15**) and can be difficult to see endoscopically.[25] The etiology of this diverticulum may be traction, owing to

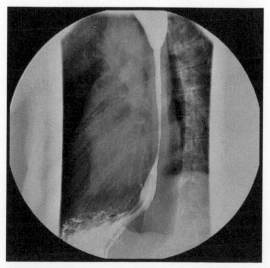

Fig. 13. Nasogastric tube stricture.

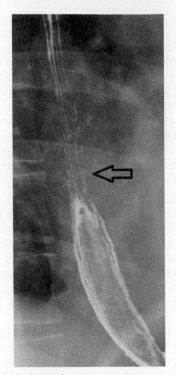

Fig. 14. Intramural diverticulosis (*arrow*).

periesophageal inflammatory lymph node disease or pulsion, presumably owing to an esophageal motor disorder, although not necessarily achalasia. Traction diverticula tend to present with a more tethered appearance with a wider opening when compared with a pulsion diverticulum.

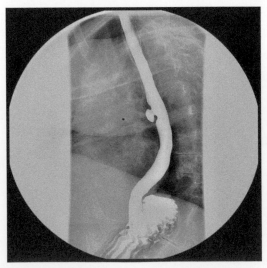

Fig. 15. Mid esophageal pulsion diverticulum.

USE OF BARIUM TO DESCRIBE ESOPHAGEAL PHYSIOLOGY

Although the principal of this article has discussed the role of barium esophagography in diagnosis of disease, one of the most important uses of this technique is in the elucidation of esophageal function. Specifically, by having an accurate means of visualizing bolus visualization and transit, fluoroscopy with barium used in conjunction with other means of measuring esophageal motility has become a cornerstone of the foundation of understanding normal and abnormal esophageal motility. For example, several of the fundamental findings of esophageal motility using these techniques simultaneously include the following: (1) establishing a 30-mm Hg contraction amplitude as the cutoff for ineffective bolus transit; (2) the timing of bolus transport with the onset of the contractile wave rather than the peak; (3) the timing of peristalsis with pharyngeal contraction; (4) peristaltic velocity; (5) the effect of bolus consistency on peristaltic function, and (6) the physiology of gastroesophageal junction opening.

Video esophagography has also elucidated many if not most of the mechanisms of oropharyngeal swallowing function. Examples include the following: (1) The role of tongue motion in bolus propulsion; (2) the role of pharyngeal contraction in bolus clearance; (3) coordination of opening, closing, and elevation of the upper esophageal sphincter with swallowing, and with concordant manometry, and (4) correlations of high intrabolus pressures with upper esophageal sphincter relaxation and opening.

Needless to say, it is with the description of these normal physiologic events using esophageal radiography with or without simultaneous manometry that has helped to define many of the esophageal dysmotility disorders.

SUMMARY

Barium esophagography, although an old test, remains important to the understanding of esophageal physiology and diagnosis of esophageal disorders. It is valuable in giving additive and/or confirmatory information to endoscopy and is the more accurate means of yielding the diagnosis. Barium esophagography also has the distinct advantages of allowing the clinician to correlate symptoms with barium findings, particularly during fluoroscopy and with varied textures substances. It also allows, particularly for oropharyngeal dysfunction, an ability to implement therapeutic maneuvers and instructions while testing. The caveat to maintaining the benefits of barium esophagography is continuing to promote and support expertise from our radiologists in performing these studies, which has been challenged by our cost-efficient and high-tech medical society.

REFERENCES

1. Levine MS, Rubesin SE, Herlinger H, et al. Double-contrast upper gastrointestinal examination: technique and interpretation. Radiology 1988;168:593–602.
2. Kahrilas PJ, Dodds WJ, Hogan WJ. Effect of peristaltic dysfunction on esophageal volume clearance. Gastroenterology 1988;94:73–80.
3. Vaezi MF, Baker ME, Achkar E, et al. Timed barium oesophagram: better predictor of long term success after pneumatic dilation in achalasia than symptom assessment. Gut 2002;50:765–70.
4. Nicodeme F, Pandolfino JE, Lin Z, et al. Adding a radial dimension to the assessment of esophagogastric junction relaxation: validation studies of the 3D-eSleeve. Am J Physiol Gastrointest Liver Physiol 2012;303:G275–80.

5. Kwiatek MA, Nicodeme F, Pandolfino JE, et al. Pressure morphology of the relaxed lower esophageal sphincter: the formation and collapse of the phrenic ampulla. Am J Physiol Gastrointest Liver Physiol 2012;302:G389–96.

6. Kahrilas PJ, Lin S, Chen J, et al. The effect of hiatus hernia on gastro-oesophageal junction pressure. Gut 1999;44:476–82.

7. Kahrilas PJ, Lin S, Chen J, et al. Oropharyngeal accommodation to swallow volume. Gastroenterology 1996;111:297–306.

8. Pikus L, Levine MS, Yang YX, et al. Videofluoroscopic studies of swallowing dysfunction and the relative risk of pneumonia. AJR Am J Roentgenol 2003;180:1613–6.

9. Law R, Katzka DA, Baron TH. Zenker's diverticulum. Clin Gastroenterol Hepatol 2013. [Epub ahead of print].

10. Rubesin SE, Levine MS. Killian-Jamieson diverticula: radiographic findings in 16 patients. AJR Am J Roentgenol 2001;177:85–9.

11. Fiorentino E, Matranga D, Pantuso G, et al. Accuracy of the water-siphon test associated to barium study in a high prevalence gastro-oesophageal reflux disease population: a novel statistical approach. J Eval Clin Pract 2010;16:550–5.

12. Pan JJ, Levine MS, Redfern RO, et al. Gastroesophageal reflux: comparison of barium studies with 24-h pH monitoring. Eur J Radiol 2003;47:149–53.

13. Ott DJ, Chen YM, Wu WC, et al. Radiographic and endoscopic sensitivity in detecting lower esophageal mucosal ring. AJR Am J Roentgenol 1986;147:261–5.

14. Davis CS, Baldea A, Johns JR, et al. The evolution and long-term results of laparoscopic antireflux surgery for the treatment of gastroesophageal reflux disease. JSLS 2010;14:332–41.

15. Vaezi MF, Pandolfino JE, Vela MF. ACG clinical guideline: diagnosis and management of achalasia. Am J Gastroenterol 2013;108:1238–49 [quiz: 1250].

16. Nicodeme F, de Ruigh A, Xiao Y, et al. A comparison of symptom severity and bolus retention with Chicago classification esophageal pressure topography metrics in patients with achalasia. Clin Gastroenterol Hepatol 2013;11:131–7 [quiz: e15].

17. Oezcelik A, Hagen JA, Halls JM, et al. An improved method of assessing esophageal emptying using the timed barium study following surgical myotomy for achalasia. J Gastrointest Surg 2009;13:14–8.

18. Muller S, Puhl S, Vieth M, et al. Analysis of symptoms and endoscopic findings in 117 patients with histological diagnoses of eosinophilic esophagitis. Endoscopy 2007;39:339–44.

19. Lucendo AJ, Pascual-Turrion JM, Navarro M, et al. Endoscopic, bioptic, and manometric findings in eosinophilic esophagitis before and after steroid therapy: a case series. Endoscopy 2007;39:765–71.

20. Croese J, Fairley SK, Masson JW, et al. Clinical and endoscopic features of eosinophilic esophagitis in adults. Gastrointest Endosc 2003;58:516–22.

21. Lee J, Huprich J, Kujath C, et al. Esophageal diameter is decreased in some patients with eosinophilic esophagitis and might increase with topical corticosteroid therapy. Clin Gastroenterol Hepatol 2012;10:481–6.

22. Katzka DA, Smyrk TC, Bruce AJ, et al. Variations in presentations of esophageal involvement in lichen planus. Clin Gastroenterol Hepatol 2010;8:777–82.

23. Contini S, Scarpignato C. Caustic injury of the upper gastrointestinal tract: a comprehensive review. World J Gastroenterol 2013;19:3918–30.

24. Canon CL, Levine MS, Cherukuri R, et al. Intramural tracking: a feature of esophageal intramural pseudodiverticulosis. AJR Am J Roentgenol 2000;175:371–4.

25. Rice TW, Baker ME. Midthoracic esophageal diverticula. Semin Thorac Cardiovasc Surg 1999;11:352–7.

Ambulatory Esophageal pH Monitoring

Michelle S. Han, MD[a], Jeffrey H. Peters, MD[b],*

KEYWORDS

- Esophageal pH monitoring • Gastroesophageal reflux disease • Catheter-based
- Wireless-based • Impedance

KEY POINTS

- Physicians should have a general knowledge of the diagnostic accuracy of each pH monitoring method.
- Prolonged pH monitoring and the combined impedance function increase the amount of information available for esophageal acid exposure evaluation; however, their effects on gastroesophageal reflux disease (GERD) diagnosis and clinical management are still under ongoing investigation.
- Prolonged pH monitoring increases the reflux detection rate.
- Because of the complexity of GERD diagnosis, routine pH monitoring should be performed for patients who are undergoing evaluation for antireflux surgery.

INTRODUCTION

The first link between gastric acid and gastroesophageal reflux (GER) was reported in 1884 after the retrieval of an acid-contained sponge from the esophagus of a patient with heartburn. The association between esophageal mucosal damage and the presence of acidic juice in the esophagus slowly emerged over the early part of the twentieth century. In 1958, Tuttle and Grossman[1,2] first measured esophageal acid reflux using an existing gastric pH meter with manometry. Johnson and DeMeester[1] established the foundation of esophageal pH monitoring in 1974 after studying GER in normal subjects and patients with reflux symptoms. In this landmark study, not only the methodology of esophageal pH monitoring and the normal reference values were defined but also a composite scoring system, the DeMeester score, was created to quantify acid exposure using 6 pH parameters.[1] This scoring system has been widely validated and is used today. With the advancement of technology, the sponge was replaced by glass and then antimony electrode catheters and in the 1990s to a

Disclosure: Nothing to disclose.
[a] Department of Surgery, University of Rochester Medical Center, University of Rochester, 601 Elmwood Avenue, Box SURG, Rochester, NY 14642, USA; [b] Department of Surgery, University Hospitals, 11100 Euclid Avenue, Cleveland, OH 44106, USA
* Corresponding author.
E-mail address: jeffrey.peters@UHhospitals.org

wireless implantable capsule; but the concept of esophageal pH monitoring for the evaluation of GER disease (GERD) has not changed over the past hundred years. The aims of this article are to review the current methods of ambulatory esophageal pH monitoring, compare the advantage and disadvantage of each test, and to discuss current controversies of each method in an effort to elucidate future directions in the diagnosis of GERD.

ESOPHAGEAL pH MONITORING: WHAT, WHY, AND WHEN

Esophageal pH monitoring is a direct in vivo measurement of esophageal acid exposure over time for the evaluation of GERD. It can be currently performed using either catheter-based or wireless systems (**Fig. 1**). Catheter-based pH monitoring requires transnasal placement of the catheter, with its measuring electrode located 5 cm above the manometrically measured upper border of lower esophageal sphincter (LES). A wireless-based pH capsule is generally placed endoscopically, 6 cm above the squamocolumnar junction (SCJ), or in the setting of Barrett esophagus above the top of the gastric rugal folds. The pH recordings of 24 hours, 48 hours, or 96 hours are currently possible, depending on the choice of device (catheter vs wireless), patient tolerability, and the duration a capsule remains attached. In the case of wireless monitoring, the pH data (sampled at a frequency of once every 6 seconds) are transmitted to an external radiofrequency recorder and then transferred to a computer with commercial software allowing automatic and/or manual analysis. Patients are generally asked to keep a diary recording symptoms, body positions, and meal periods during the time of pH monitoring allowing the analysis of reflux patterns and symptom correlation measures. **Fig. 2** demonstrates the basic steps of the test. Currently available and widely used pH monitoring options are listed in **Box 1**.

Esophageal pH monitoring is a crucial part of GERD evaluation. According to the 2007 American College of Gastroenterology's practice guidelines for esophageal reflux testing, pH monitoring

1. Is useful in documenting abnormal esophageal reflux exposure in endoscopy-negative patients with typical reflux symptoms who failed medical therapy and are being considered for antireflux surgery

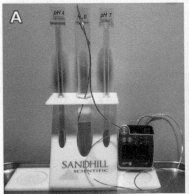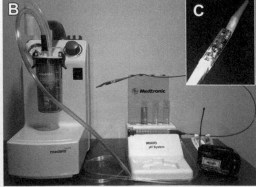

Fig. 1. Ambulatory esophageal pH monitoring: catheter-based (*A*) or wireless-based device (*B*; Bravo, Given Imaging Ltd, Yoqneam, Israel). The Bravo capsule (*C*) is loaded on the delivery system. (Images used with permission from Medtronic, Minneapolis, MN; Sandhill Scientific, Highlands Ranch, CO; Medela Inc, McHenry, IL; and Given Imaging, a Covidien company. The use of any Covidien photo or image does not imply Covidien review or endorsement of any article or publication.)

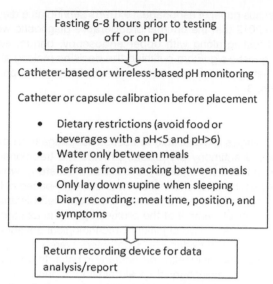

Fig. 2. Basic steps of ambulatory esophageal pH monitoring. PPI, proton pump inhibitor.

2. May be useful in detecting the adequacy of acid control in patients with Barrett esophagus, atypical reflux symptoms, or recurrent symptoms after antireflux surgery[3]
3. May be useful when combined with impedance in detecting nonacid reflux or in evaluating patients whose reflux symptoms are not controlled by a proton pump inhibitor (PPI; PPI nonresponders)[3]

Patients presenting with typical reflux symptoms are given the diagnosis of GERD liberally by health care providers from many specialties. Studies have shown that symptoms, reflux or hiatal hernia detected by barium esophagram, and even findings of mucosal injury on endoscopy are either unreliable or not sensitive in diagnosing GERD; thus, esophageal pH monitoring becomes an integral part of the diagnostic and treatment plan.[4] The Diamond study, a single-blind prospective study of 308 patients published in 2010, concluded that the Reflux Disease Questionnaire, family practitioners, and gastroenterologists all had similar diagnostic accuracy for GERD (sensitivity 62%–67%; specificity 63%–70%). In this study, the 48-hour Bravo (Given Imaging Ltd, Yoqneam, Israel) pH-monitoring result, endoscopic findings of esophagitis, symptom association probability (SAP) of 95% or more, or the borderline pH-monitoring result with response to PPI therapy were used as the gold standard for

---

Box 1
Available pH-monitoring tests

Catheter based (transnasal placement at 5 cm above upper border of LES)

• Conventional 24-hour catheter pH monitoring; dual-channel pH monitoring

• 24-hour multichannel intraluminal impedance pH monitoring

Wireless based (endoscopic placement at 6 cm above SCJ)

• 48-hour Bravo (Given Imaging Ltd, Yoqneam, Israel) pH monitoring

• 96-hour Bravo pH monitoring

diagnosis. A consensus panel of esophageal experts serving as a diagnostic advisory panel concluded in 2012 that the optimal preoperative diagnostic workup for GERD should include pH testing along with upper endoscopy, barium esophagram, and manometry.[5] A diagnostic algorithm outlining the decision making and test selection process when evaluating patients suspected to have abnormal esophageal acid exposure is shown in **Fig. 3**.

TEST SELECTION

A variety of methodologies are available to assess esophageal pH exposure. Single-sensor catheter-based antimony pH probes provide the traditional and heretofore most widely used method. Conventionally, this is a 24-hour study, which detects distal esophageal acid exposure. Dual-channel 24-hour catheter-based pH monitoring provides data on proximal esophageal exposure, although fixed distances between the pH sensors results in misplacement of the proximal probe in as many as 45% of patients, limiting its usefulness.[6] Two significant technological advances were made in the 1990s. First, combined impedance-pH catheters were developed, allowing the assessment of the role of nonacid reflux particularly in patients with atypical and/or refractory reflux symptoms (multichannel intraluminal impedance pH monitoring [MII-pH], **Fig. 4A**). Second, wireless implantable pH sensors were developed, allowing ambulatory recording of 48 hours and now up to 96 hours in the absence of a transnasal catheter (see **Fig. 4B**). The investigators recommend that patients with typical GERD symptoms, such as heartburn and regurgitation, should undergo at least a conventional pH study given the poor sensitivity and specificity of symptom-based diagnosis of GERD.[7] In contrast to common belief, a trial of PPI for symptom response does not improve the diagnostic accuracy.[8] The optimal strategy for test selection

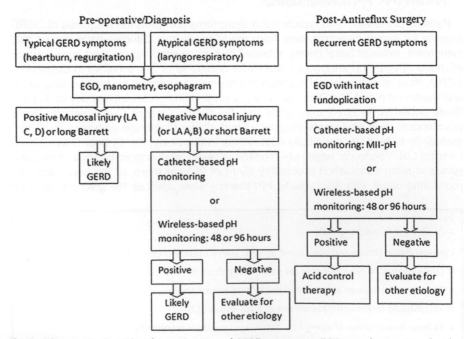

Fig. 3. Diagnostic algorithm for evaluation of GERD symptoms. EGD, esophagogastroduodenoscopy; LA, Los Angeles.

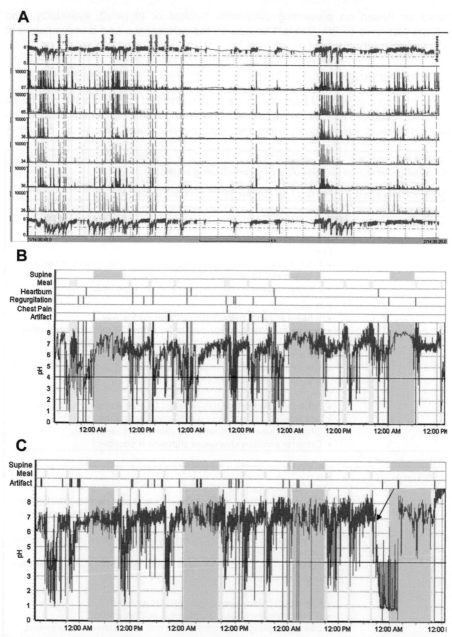

Fig. 4. (*A*) Ambulatory 24-hour MII-pH monitoring: pH tracing. (*B*) pH tracing (96-hour Bravo pH monitoring). Patient positions, meal period, and symptoms are marked along the recording time line. (*C*) The pH tracing showing premature dislodgement of the Bravo capsule on day 4. The pH decreased abruptly to pH less than 1 (*arrow*) and then recovered to pH greater than 8.

should be based on presenting symptoms (typical or atypical), availability, and perhaps response to PPI. **Table 1** compares the advantages and disadvantages of each testing method.

TEST INTERPRETATION

All patients who undergo pH monitoring are required to fast 6 to 8 hours and to be off antacid medications for 5 to 7 days before catheter or capsule placement. On-therapy (stay on antacid medications) tests can also be done and are most commonly

Table 1 Comparison of the current ambulatory pH monitoring methods	
pH-Monitoring Test	**Pro and Con for Test Selection Consideration**
Catheter-based	
24-h conventional	Pro • It has transnasal placement without endoscopy. Con • Patient discomfort causes reduced oral intake or daily activity. • It only measures distal esophageal acid exposure. • Catheter position change and slippage is possible.
MII-pH	Pro • It has transnasal placement without endoscopy. • It detects nonacid reflux and bolus transit. It may provide useful information in patients with atypical symptoms, nonacid reflux, or refractory reflux symptoms. • The multichannel can measure acid and nonacid reflux both distal and proximally. Con • Patient discomfort causes reduced oral intake or daily activity. • Test results may not necessarily alter the management plan. Ongoing research is needed to validate its usefulness. • Catheter position change or slippage is possible.
Wireless-based	
48-h Bravo	Pro • It eliminates patient discomfort. • The capsule is fixed eliminating concerns of movement or slippage. • It is more physiologic and has minimal effects on daily activity or oral intake. • Longer duration of monitoring is possible with an increased reflux detection rate. • Passage with bowel movement eliminates additional clinic visit for catheter removal. Con • Endoscopic placement might require sedation. • it only measures distal esophageal acid exposure. • Lower sampling frequency might not detect short reflux events. • Premature capsule dislodgement could occur. • A rare case with severe discomfort might require endoscopic removal.
96-h Bravo	Pro • They are the same as above. In addition, prolonged duration of monitoring might increase the reflux detection rate further. There is improved sensitivity with high specificity. Con • They are the same as above.

performed on patients who have refractory reflux symptoms.[3] The widely accepted cutoff of a pH less than 4 defining a reflux episode is from Tuttle and colleagues'[9] original work in 1961. It is based on the fact that the onset of pyrosis was induced when the distal esophagus was exposed to acidic fluid perfusion at a pH less than 4[9] and the acidic acid dissociation constant (pKa) of pepsin. Many recommend dietary restrictions, although further studies are needed to evaluate its effect on pH monitoring results.[10] Parameters reported are listed in **Box 2**. Published normal values for the catheter-based and wireless systems are summarized in **Table 2**.

Fig. 5 outlines the brief steps for test interpretation. All pH-monitoring tests provide information on distal esophageal acid exposure, the patterns of reflux, and symptom correlation measures. Monitoring pH with impedance (MII-pH) has the added ability to evaluate bolus transit of gas or liquid and nonacid reflux. A pH less than 4 is the widely accepted cutoff to denote an acid reflux episode. A percent time greater than 5 or DeMeester score greater than 14.72 is used to define a positive study. Wireless tests provide longer duration of monitoring: 48 to 96 hours. The capsule, on average, detaches 5 to 7 days after placement. The success rates (complete data acquisition without premature detachment) for a 48-hour and 96-hour pH recording are 90% and 41% to 90%, respectively.[11–14] Premature capsule dislodgement can be easily identified on the pH tracing with an abrupt decrease of pH to less than 2 (gastric pH) for 3 to 4 hours followed by a recovery of pH to more than 8 (intestinal pH) (see **Fig. 4**C). It is important to recognize premature capsule dislodgement because the software-generated pH parameters, DeMeester scores, and symptom correlation measures would be falsely elevated. The wireless test can be interpreted using the average 48-hour or 96-hour data or the worst-day data. Studies suggest that defining abnormality using the worst-day data is more sensitive,[3] which concurs with the known day-to-day variation in reflux patterns in both health and disease.[15,16]

The 24-hour MII-pH test measures both esophageal impedance and distal esophageal acid exposure (**Fig. 6**). The detection of upward retrograde impedance change (gas or liquid) without a pH decrease to less than 4 is defined as a nonacid reflux event. Nonacid events are further divided into weakly acidic reflux (pH 4.0–6.9) or alkaline reflux (pH≥7). Impedance data of the proximal and distal esophagus can provide information on the height of reflux and the type of refluxate.

Box 2
pH parameters reported by pH-monitoring test

- Total percent time of pH less than 4
- Percent time of pH less than 4 in upright position
- Percent time of pH less than 4 in supine position
- Total number of reflux episodes (pH<4)
- Number of reflux episodes greater than 5 minutes
- Duration of the longest reflux episode
- Calculated DeMeester score
- Total test duration, test duration in upright and supine position, and in postprandial period
- Symptom correlation measures (symptom index, symptom sensitivity index, symptom association probability)
- The complete pH tracing (see **Fig. 4**)
- Impedance data (MII-pH test only)

Table 2
Summary of normal values for each method of pH monitoring (values are 95th percentiles)

Catheter-Based	Johnson & DeMeester[1,a]	Jamieson et al[32]	Richter et al[33]
Total time pH <4 (%)	4.2	4.5	5.78
Upright time pH <4 (%)	6.3	8.4	8.15
Supine time pH <4 (%)	1.2	3.5	3.45
No. of reflux episodes	50.0	46.9	46.0
No. of reflux episodes ≥5 min	3.0	3.5	4.0
Longest episode (min)	9.2	19.8	18.45

MII-pH		Shay et al[34]	Zerbib et al[35]
Total time pH <4 (%)		6.3	5.0
Upright time pH <4 (%)		9.7	6.2
Supine time pH <4 (%)		2.1	5.3
No. of total reflux episodes		73	75
No. of acid reflux episodes		55	50
No. of weakly acid reflux episodes		26	33
No. of non-acid reflux episodes		1	15
Total bolus exposure (%)		1.4	2.0
Upright bolus exposure (%)		9.7	2.7
Supine bolus exposure (%)		2.1	0.9

Wireless-Based[b]	First 24 h	Second 24 h	Combined
Total time pH <4 (%)	6.31	5.87	4.85
Upright time pH <4 (%)	7.99	7.47	7.29
Supine time pH <4 (%)	1.60	1.33	1.39
No. of reflux episodes	58	60	104
No. of reflux episodes ≥5 min	4	3	5
Longest episode (min)	12.24	19.48	16.18
DeMeester score	17.95	15.76	14.98

[a] Values are Mean ± 2 SD.
[b] *Data from* Ayazi S, Lipham JC, Portale G, et al. Bravo catheter-free pH monitoring: normal values, concordance, optimal diagnostic thresholds, and accuracy. Clin Gastroenterol Hepatol 2009;7(1):60–7.

Three clinically distinct patterns of pathologic reflux were described by DeMeester in 1976 and include upright, supine, and combined (bipositional).[17] In this landmark study, the severity of symptoms and physiologic defects were associated with reflux patterns.

Symptom correlation measures provide potentially meaningful associations between symptoms and reflux events. As stated before, pH monitoring only demonstrates distal esophageal acid exposure; judgment is required to conclude that it is the cause of symptoms. Symptom index (SI), symptom sensitivity index (SSI), and symptom association probability (SAP) have been proposed as clinically useful tools to assess how a particular symptom is associated with detected reflux events. Among the 3 measures, it is generally thought that the SAP is most statistically valid[3]; few symptoms other than heartburn have received any meaningful study. Their usefulness in the clinical management of GERD remains an area of investigation. **Box 3** lists the calculation formulas and statistical consideration for each index.

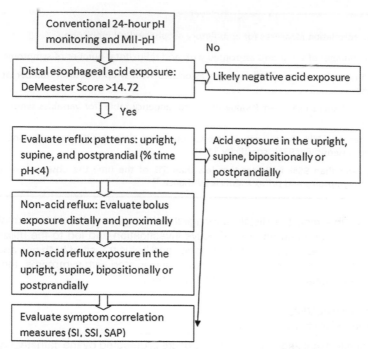

Fig. 5. Test interpretation steps for pH monitoring. SAP, symptom association probability; SI, symptom index; SSI, symptom sensitivity index.

When interpreting test results, it is critically important to know the diagnostic accuracy (sensitivity, specificity, positive predictive value, negative predictive value) of the individual test (**Table 3**). A negative pH-monitoring result does not mean that the patient does not have GERD. It only demonstrates that, with the intrinsic diagnostic

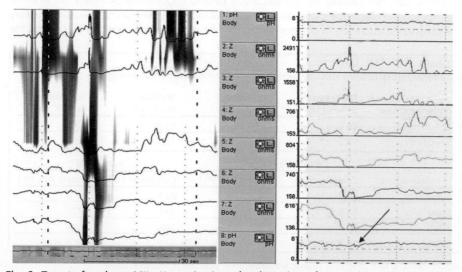

Fig. 6. Twenty-four-hour MII-pH monitoring: the detection of upward impedance change (*left*) without a pH decrease less than 4 (*right, arrow*) is defined as a nonacid reflux event.

Box 3
Symptom correlation measures for ambulatory esophageal pH monitoring

- SI is the number of symptoms associated with acid reflux/total number of symptoms.
- SSI is the total number of reflux events associated with symptoms/total number of reflux episodes.
- SAP is the Fisher's exact test *P* value of the contingency table (for variables symptom and reflux).
- SI greater than 50% is the optimal receiver operating characteristic curve threshold for a positive SI (sensitivity 93%, specificity 71%).
- SAP greater than 95% indicates that less than 5% of the time the observed association between symptoms and reflux events is by chance.[41]

---

accuracy of this test, the distal esophageal acid exposure is within normal limits. Nonacid reflux has been an area of active investigation and led to the utilization of impedance to detect nonacid reflux episodes and bolus transit of both gas and liquid; however, at the current time, although clearly associated with symptoms, the clinical implications of nonacid reflux warrant further study.

CURRENT CONTROVERSIES
pH Electrode Placement Location

Conventionally distal esophageal acid exposure is detected by the catheter tip placed at 5 cm above the upper border of the LES or the Bravo capsule located at 6 cm above the SCJ. Both the catheter and capsule position have been areas of investigation. Pandolfino and colleagues[18] compared wireless and catheter-based systems, measuring the tip and the capsule position via fluoroscopy immediately after placement. The mean absolute difference in position between the two systems was 1.0 cm, and the two placement methods resulted in similar tip and capsule positions. More importantly, they showed that the difference in acid exposure between the two systems was not caused by the electrode position. Controversy exists on whether positioning the electrode closer to the gastroesophageal (GE) junction would increase the diagnostic accuracy of pH monitoring.[19,20] Studies have shown that by placing the

---

Table 3
Summary of sensitivity and specificity for each method of pH monitoring

Catheter-Based[a]	DeMeester et al[37] (%)	Johnsson et al[38] (%)	Mattioli et al[39] (%)	Schindlbeck et al[40,b] (%)
Sensitivity	88.0	87.0	85.0	93.3
Specificity	73.0	97.0	100	92.9

	Pandolfino et al[14]		Ayazi et al[36]	
Wireless-Based	**Combined (%)**	**Worst Day (%)**	**Combined (%)**	**Worst Day (%)**
Sensitivity	64.9	83.8	82.0	93.0
Specificity	94.8	84.5	100	100
PPV	92.3	83.8	100	100
NPV	74.0	84.6	67.0	83.0

Abbreviations: NPV, negative predictive value; PPV, positive predictive value.
[a] Ambulatory 24-hour intraesophageal pH monitoring only.
[b] Only percent time of pH less than 4 is considered.

electrodes closer to the LES than the conventional 5 cm above measures higher acid exposure.[21,22] Wenner and colleagues[19] compared the diagnostic performance between standard electrode placement and a position 1 cm above the SCJ. They reported an increase in test sensitivity from 63% to 86% in patients either with or without esophagitis. A similar study comparing the measurement of acid reflux 1 cm above the gastroesophageal junction to 5 cm showed improved diagnostic accuracy in patients with erosive esophagitis but not in patients with nonerosive reflux disease.[20] Although there is not sufficient evidence to recommend more proximal placement in current clinical practice, the possibility that diagnostic accuracy would be improved by an alternate electrode placement is real and may help explain patients with functional heartburn or those with endoscopic findings of short-segment Barrett esophagus but a negative pH-monitoring result.

Discrepancy Between the Two Systems

Simultaneous catheter-based and Bravo pH monitoring has been conducted over the years to allow comparisons of the two methodologies. In general, studies have reported a higher acid exposure measured by the catheter system comparing with the wireless-based system, although the reasons are largely unclear. Sampling rates may be a cause of discrepancy. Sampling frequency is 4 per second for most catheter-based systems, whereas it is every 6 seconds for the Bravo system, a considerable difference. Des Varannes and colleagues[23] reported significant correlation in acid exposure between the two systems (r = 0.87) and concluded that although the Bravo system under recorded acid exposure, its ability to prolong recording time significantly improved the sensitivity of pH monitoring for the diagnosis of GERD. Pandolfino and colleagues[18] also reported lower acid exposure measurements with the Bravo system. They suggested that electrode thermal calibration and pH drift are potential causes of discrepancy between the two systems. The use of an in vivo pH reference (orange juice) was able to improve the discrepancy between the pH data sets of the two systems. A Swedish study simultaneously comparing the two systems reported similar underestimation of acid exposure by the Bravo system and concluded that the two systems are not interchangeable in practice.[24]

With the added ability to measure bolus transit, reflux height, and nonacid reflux events, MII-pH has been preferentially used to evaluate patients with atypical GERD symptoms, such as laryngo-respiratory symptoms or refractory GERD symptoms (PPI nonresponders). A retrospective review of 66 patients, most with atypical reflux symptoms, who underwent both MII-pH and Bravo pH monitoring at the University of Rochester found that 44% of the patients had discordant results. Of these, 90% had a negative MII-pH but positive Bravo study. The authors concluded that a single 24-hour MII-pH study may be an inadequate test to exclude GERD in this patient population. Prakash and Clouse[25] also reported that the prolonged recording time of the Bravo system increases the reflux detection rate, especially in patients with atypical symptoms. More investigations are needed to study the discrepancies between the two systems in order to make sound clinical recommendations for the clinical utility of each system.

The Influence of Diet on Test Accuracy

Although dietary guidelines are generally not given when pH monitoring is performed, studies have shown that exclusion of the meal period would remove the effects of acidic food ingestion and improve the diagnostic accuracy.[14,26,27] Studies have suggested that 5 minutes of acidic food ingestion has a significant effect on the outcome of pH monitoring.[10] There are no current clinical guidelines on whether or not diet restrictions should be given, and the current preference likely varies among centers and clinics.

On or Off PPI Therapy

A recent diagnostic algorithm for esophageal disorders suggested by Kahrilas and Smout[28] supported the role of a PPI trial as an integral part of the diagnostic workup for GERD. The controversy lies when and if PPIs should be continued during pH monitoring. Most reports have shown that symptomatic PPI nonresponders usually have normal results on pH monitoring.[29] Most experts think that pH monitoring should be performed off PPI therapy to optimize the chance of detecting reflux events.[30,31] Garrean and colleagues[11] combined 48 hours on and off PPI therapy using 96-hour Bravo pH monitoring and reported enhanced test interpretation. According to the American College of Gastroenterology's practice guideline in 2007, testing off therapy is recommended to rule out GERD, whereas on-therapy testing is used to evaluate refractory GERD symptoms.[3] A positive pH-monitoring test of the later scenario suggests that more aggressive therapy or other management plans might be needed.

SUMMARY AND FUTURE DIRECTIONS

- Esophageal pH monitoring is an integral part of the diagnostic workup for GERD.
- There are 2 major systems: the catheter-based or the wireless-based Bravo pH monitoring. All pH monitoring demonstrates distal esophageal acid exposure. MII-pH, in addition, can evaluate bolus transit, reflux height, and nonacid reflux events. Prolonged wireless pH monitoring increases the reflux detection rate and may be the test of choice to evaluate patients with atypical symptoms or PPI nonresponders.
- Test selection should be based on availability, patient symptoms (typical or atypical), and the response to the PPI trial to optimize diagnostic accuracy.
- Test interpretation includes the following: distal esophageal acid exposure, patterns of reflux, inclusion or exclusion of the meal period, impedance (nonacid reflux), and symptom correlation measures (SI, SSI, SAP).
- Monitoring pH, although not perfect, is the single most useful diagnostic test for GERD evaluation. For patients with typical GERD symptoms who are endoscopy-negative, a pH-monitoring test is required for consideration of antireflux surgery. A positive pH study predicts relief of typical symptoms postoperatively.
- Prolonged wireless pH monitoring and possibly a smaller capsule that is placed closer to the GE junction than the conventional position may be useful future advances to improve the diagnosis of GERD.

REFERENCES

1. Johnson LF, Demeester TR. Twenty-four-hour pH monitoring of the distal esophagus. A quantitative measure of gastroesophageal reflux. Am J Gastroenterol 1974;62(4):325–32.
2. Herbella FA, Nipominick I, Patti MG. From sponges to capsules. The history of esophageal pH monitoring. Dis Esophagus 2009;22(2):99–103.
3. Hirano I, Richter JE. ACG practice guidelines: esophageal reflux testing. Am J Gastroenterol 2007;102(3):668–85.
4. Bello B, Zoccali M, Gullo R, et al. Gastroesophageal reflux disease and antireflux surgery-what is the proper preoperative work-up? J Gastrointest Surg 2013;17(1): 14–20 [discussion: p20].

5. Jobe BA, Richter JE, Hoppo T, et al. Preoperative diagnostic workup before anti-reflux surgery: an evidence and experience-based consensus of the Esophageal Diagnostic Advisory Panel. J Am Coll Surg 2013;217(4):586–97.

6. McCollough M, Jabbar A, Cacchione R, et al. Proximal sensor data from routine dual-sensor esophageal pH monitoring is often inaccurate. Dig Dis Sci 2004; 49(10):1607–11.

7. Dent J, Vakil N, Jones R, et al. Accuracy of the diagnosis of GORD by question-naire, physicians and a trial of proton pump inhibitor treatment: the Diamond Study. Gut 2010;59(6):714–21.

8. Bytzer P, Jones R, Vakil N, et al. Limited ability of the proton-pump inhibitor test to identify patients with gastroesophageal reflux disease. Clin Gastroenterol Hepatol 2012;10(12):1360–6.

9. Tuttle SG, Rufin F, Bettarello A. The physiology of heartburn. Ann Intern Med 1961;55:292–300.

10. Koskenvuo JW, Parkka JP, Hartiala JJ, et al. Ingested acidic food and liquids may lead to misinterpretation of 24-hour ambulatory pH tests: focus on measurement of extra-esophageal reflux. Dig Dis Sci 2007;52(7):1678–84.

11. Garrean CP, Zhang Q, Gonsalves N, et al. Acid reflux detection and symptom-reflux association using 4-day wireless pH recording combining 48-hour periods off and on PPI therapy. Am J Gastroenterol 2008;103(7):1631–7.

12. Grigolon A, Consonni D, Bravi I, et al. Diagnostic yield of 96-h wireless pH moni-toring and usefulness in patients' management. Scand J Gastroenterol 2011; 46(5):522–30.

13. Scarpulla G, Camilleri S, Galante P, et al. The impact of prolonged pH measure-ments on the diagnosis of gastroesophageal reflux disease: 4-day wireless pH studies. Am J Gastroenterol 2007;102(12):2642–7.

14. Pandolfino JE, Richter JE, Ours T, et al. Ambulatory esophageal pH monitoring using a wireless system. Am J Gastroenterol 2003;98(4):740–9.

15. Ayazi S, Hagen JA, Zehetner J, et al. Day-to-day discrepancy in Bravo pH moni-toring is related to the degree of deterioration of the lower esophageal sphincter and severity of reflux disease. Surg Endosc 2011;25(7):2219–23.

16. Ahlawat SK, Novak DJ, Williams DC, et al. Day-to-day variability in acid reflux pat-terns using the BRAVO pH monitoring system. J Clin Gastroenterol 2006;40(1):20–4.

17. Demeester TR, Johnson LF, Joseph GJ, et al. Patterns of gastroesophageal reflux in health and disease. Ann Surg 1976;184(4):459–70.

18. Pandolfino JE, Schreiner MA, Lee TJ, et al. Comparison of the Bravo wireless and Digitrapper catheter-based pH monitoring systems for measuring esophageal acid exposure. Am J Gastroenterol 2005;100(7):1466–76.

19. Wenner J, Hall M, Hoglund P, et al. Wireless pH recording immediately above the squamocolumnar junction improves the diagnostic performance of esophageal pH studies. Am J Gastroenterol 2008;103(12):2977–85.

20. Bansal A, Wani S, Rastogi A, et al. Impact of measurement of esophageal acid exposure close to the gastroesophageal junction on diagnostic accuracy and event-symptom correlation: a prospective study using wireless dual pH moni-toring. Am J Gastroenterol 2009;104(12):2918–25.

21. Mekapati J, Knight LC, Maurer AH, et al. Transsphincteric pH profile at the gastro-esophageal junction. Clin Gastroenterol Hepatol 2008;6(6):630–4.

22. Wenner J, Johnsson F, Johansson J, et al. Acid reflux immediately above the squamocolumnar junction and in the distal esophagus: simultaneous pH moni-toring using the wireless capsule pH system. Am J Gastroenterol 2006;101(8): 1734–41.

23. des Varannes SB, Mion F, Ducrotte P, et al. Simultaneous recordings of oesophageal acid exposure with conventional pH monitoring and a wireless system (Bravo). Gut 2005;54(12):1682–6.
24. Hakanson BS, Berggren P, Granqvist S, et al. Comparison of wireless 48-h (Bravo) versus traditional ambulatory 24-h esophageal pH monitoring. Scand J Gastroenterol 2009;44(3):276–83.
25. Prakash C, Clouse RE. Value of extended recording time with wireless pH monitoring in evaluating gastroesophageal reflux disease. Clin Gastroenterol Hepatol 2005;3(4):329–34.
26. Dhiman RK, Saraswat VA, Naik SR. Ambulatory esophageal pH monitoring: technique, interpretations, and clinical indications. Dig Dis Sci 2002;47(2):241–50.
27. Smout AJ. pH testing: the basics. J Clin Gastroenterol 2008;42(5):564–70.
28. Kahrilas PJ, Smout AJ. Esophageal disorders. Am J Gastroenterol 2010;105(4): 747–56.
29. Charbel S, Khandwala F, Vaezi MF. The role of esophageal pH monitoring in symptomatic patients on PPI therapy. Am J Gastroenterol 2005;100(2):283–9.
30. Hemmink GJ, Bredenoord AJ, Weusten BL, et al. Esophageal pH-impedance monitoring in patients with therapy-resistant reflux symptoms: 'on' or 'off' proton pump inhibitor? Am J Gastroenterol 2008;103(10):2446–53.
31. Kushnir VM, Sayuk GS, Gyawali CP. The effect of antisecretory therapy and study duration on ambulatory esophageal pH monitoring. Dig Dis Sci 2011;56(5): 1412–9.
32. Jamieson JR, Stein HJ, DeMeester TR, et al. Ambulatory 24-h esophageal pH monitoring: normal values, optimal thresholds, specificity, sensitivity, and reproducibility. Am J Gastroenterol 1992;87(9):1102–11.
33. Richter JE, Bradley LA, DeMeester TR, et al. Normal 24-hr ambulatory esophageal pH values. Influence of study center, pH electrode, age, and gender. Dig Dis Sci 1992;37(6):849–56.
34. Shay S, Tutuian R, Sifrim D, et al. Twenty-four hour ambulatory simultaneous impedance and pH monitoring: a multicenter report of normal values from 60 healthy volunteers. Am J Gastroenterol 2004;99(6):1037–43.
35. Zerbib F, des Varannes SB, Roman S, et al. Normal values and day-to-day variability of 24-h ambulatory oesophageal impedance-pH monitoring in a Belgian-French cohort of healthy subjects. Aliment Pharmacol Ther 2005;22(10):1011–21.
36. Ayazi S, Lipham JC, Portale G, et al. Bravo catheter-free pH monitoring: normal values, concordance, optimal diagnostic thresholds, and accuracy. Clin Gastroenterol Hepatol 2009;7(1):60–7.
37. DeMeester TR, Wang CI, Wernly JA, et al. Technique, indications, and clinical use of 24 hour esophageal pH monitoring. J Thorac Cardiovasc Surg 1980;79(5): 656–70.
38. Johnsson F, Joelsson B, Isberg PE. Ambulatory 24 hour intraesophageal pH-monitoring in the diagnosis of gastroesophageal reflux disease. Gut 1987; 28(9):1145–50.
39. Mattioli S, Pilotti V, Spangaro M, et al. Reliability of 24-hour home esophageal pH monitoring in diagnosis of gastroesophageal reflux. Dig Dis Sci 1989;34(1):71–8.
40. Schindlbeck NE, Heinrich C, Konig A, et al. Optimal thresholds, sensitivity, and specificity of long-term pH-metry for the detection of gastroesophageal reflux disease. Gastroenterology 1987;93(1):85–90.
41. Singh S, Richter JE, Bradley LA, et al. The symptom index. Differential usefulness in suspected acid-related complaints of heartburn and chest pain. Dig Dis Sci 1993;38(8):1402–8.

Evaluating Esophageal Bolus Transit by Impedance Monitoring

Radu Tutuian, MD, PhD[a,b,*]

KEYWORDS

- Multichannel intraluminal impedance • Esophageal manometry
- High-resolution esophageal manometry • Esophageal bolus transit

KEY POINTS

- Esophageal manometry (both conventional and high-resolution) assess primarily the contractility of the tubular esophagus and relaxation of sphincters.
- Intraluminal impedance measures bolus presence and transit in the esophagus without radiation, allowing for a virtually unlimited number of observations.
- Combined impedance manometry (MII-EM) and high-resolution impedance manometry (HRiM) offer a comprehensive evaluation of the esophageal function, including esophageal motility and bolus transit.

INTRODUCTION

The function of the esophagus is transporting liquids and solids from the oropharyngeal cavity into the stomach. This is achieved by the coordinated contraction of the pharyngeal musculature, timely relaxation of the upper esophageal sphincter (UES), and esophageal peristalsis and relaxation of the lower esophageal sphincter (LES). This carefully scripted interplay of striated and smooth muscles is triggered by the cranial nerves, coordinated by a vagal and intrinsic esophageal network of neurons. A disturbance of this system leads to esophageal symptoms such as dysphagia and/or chest pain.

Testing of the esophageal function includes evaluating pharyngeal and esophageal peristalsis and relaxation of the upper and lower esophageal sphincter, as well as assessing esophageal bolus transit. Esophageal motility is quantified using esophageal manometry and in recent years more often by high-resolution manometry (HRM)

[a] Division of Gastroenterology, University Clinics of Visceral Surgery and Medicine, Bern University Hospital – Inselspital Bern, Freiburgstrasse 4, Bern 3010, Switzerland; [b] Division of Gastroenterology, Spital Region Oberaargau (SRO) – Langenthal, St. Urbanstrasse 67, Langenthal 4900, Switzerland
* Divison of Gastroenterology, Spital Region Oberaargau (SRO) – Langenthal, St. Urbanstrasse 67, Langenthal 4901, Switzerland.
E-mail address: r.tutuian@sro.ch

Gastrointest Endoscopy Clin N Am 24 (2014) 595–605
http://dx.doi.org/10.1016/j.giec.2014.06.009
1052-5157/14/$ – see front matter © 2014 Elsevier Inc. All rights reserved.

with esophageal pressure topography (EPT) representation. Esophageal bolus transit has traditionally been assessed by video fluoroscopy, a method that allows visualizing the shape and progression boluses through the esophagus. The gold standard video fluoroscopy is limited by the ionizing radiation used during testing. Thus, researchers and clinicians have been looking for alternative methods to quantify esophageal bolus transit.

One alternative to fluoroscopy in assessing esophageal bolus transit is multichannel intraluminal impedance (MII). Measuring resistance to alternating current (impedance) in the esophageal lumen MII overcomes the limitation of video fluoroscopy, allowing quantification of esophageal bolus transit for virtually an unlimited number of swallows. This article summarizes studies validating this method, establishing normal values and the application of this method in clinical research and daily practice as identified by searches in PubMed for "esophageal impedance," "multichannel intraluminal impedance," "impedance manometry," and "high-resolution impedance manometry."

VALIDATION OF IMPEDANCE MEASUREMENTS TO ASSESS ESOPHAGEAL BOLUS TRANSIT

In the early 1990s, Silny[1] at the Helmholtz Institute in Aachen, Germany, published a seminal paper describing MII as a novel technique to assesses intraluminal bolus movement by measuring changes in conductivity of the intraluminal content. This method exploits differences in electrical conductivity of the esophageal wall and its content when liquid or gas bolus passes by an pair of metal rings mounted on a catheter. The empty esophagus has a fairly stable baseline impedance of 1500 to 2000 Ohms. Subsequently, Blom and colleagues[2] reported on the correlation of changes in intraluminal impedance with bolus movement during combined video fluoroscopy and impedance studies. When liquid passes by the impedance measuring segment, the following changes[3] are observed (**Figs. 1** and **2**):

1. An initial drop in impedance when the liquid bolus enters the impedance-measuring segment, since this will enable the flow of electric current
2. A low (nadir) impedance when the liquid bolus spans across both measurement rings
3. A rise in impedance as the bolus is cleared from this segment by a peristaltic wave
4. Return to baseline

In the early 2000s, Simren and colleagues[4] further validated the ability of impedance to detect bolus movement. Considering bolus entry at a 50% drop in impedance from baseline to nadir and bolus exit at the recovery of impedance to the 50% value, Simren and colleagues[4] found a strong correlation between video fluoroscopy and impedance for measuring the time of esophageal filling ($r^2 = 0.89$; $P<.0001$) and emptying ($r^2 = 0.79$; $P<.0001$).

MII classifies swallows as having complete bolus transit if the bolus enters the proximal site and exits (ie, there is a recovery of impedance above the 50% difference from baseline to nadir) from all distal impedance-measuring segments.[5] Conversely bolus transit is defined as incomplete if impedance detects bolus retention in any of the distal channels (ie, channels situated below the transition zone). Bolus retention in the transition zone (ie, in the pressure nadir between the proximal striated and distal smooth muscles of the esophageal body) is considered acceptable (ie, not abnormal). Defining normal retention in the transition zone based on impedance measurements is difficult, because impedance cannot quantify the amount of bolus retained (ie, 1 mL or 10 mL will produce the same change in intraluminal impedance).[3]

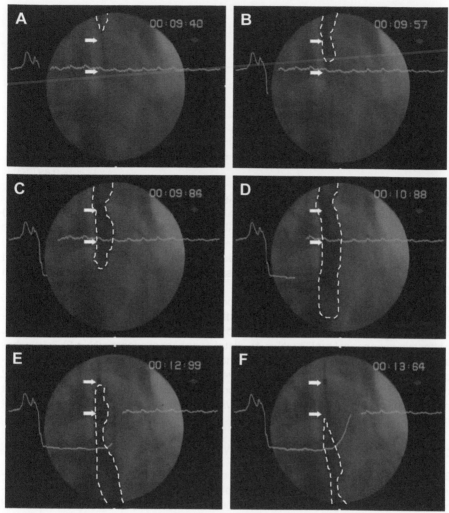

Fig. 1. Changes in intraluminal impedance as a bolus passes by the pair of impedance-measuring rings. (*A*) Esophageal baseline, bolus approaching the proximal ring. (*B*) Bolus entry characterized by a rapid drop in impedance. (*C*) Bolus passing by the distal impedance-measuring ring. (*D*) Nadir impedance as bolus is in contact with both impedance-measuring rings. (*E*) Bolus exit characterized by a rise in impedance from nadir toward baseline. (*F*) Return to esophageal baseline as the bolus has passed both impedance measuring rings. The contour of the bolus has been highlighted with a white-dashed line. The white arrows indicate the position of the impedance rings on the catheter.

These definitions were confirmed by simultaneous barium impedance and manometry studies in a group of 15 normal volunteers.[6] Imam and colleagues correlated impedance manometry findings with simultaneously recorded video fluoroscopic barium swallows in 15 normal volunteers (11 women, mean age 43 years). Fluoroscopy and impedance measurements correlated in 83 of 86 (97%) of swallows. Normal bolus transit was found in 61 of 83 swallows with normal contraction amplitude and complete bolus transit; stasis occurred in 7 of 83 swallows despite normal contraction amplitude in 4 of 7 swallows, and retrograde escape occurred in 14 of 83 swallows,

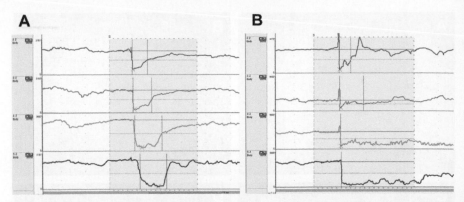

Fig. 2. Swallows evaluated by multichannel intraluminal impedance. (*A*) Swallow with complete bolus transit (bolus entry in the proximal channel and exit in all 3 distal channels). (*B*) Swallow with incomplete bolus transit (ie, failed bolus exit in the 2 distal channels).

allowing the authors to conclude that impedance monitoring is a valid transit test and describe bolus transit patterns in normal subjects for comparison with patients with esophageal motility disorders.

More recently, Cho and colleagues[7] reported on the results of concomitant multichannel intraluminal impedance and video fluoroscopy recordings in a group of 16 patients with dysphagia. This group included patients with normal manometry (N = 6), ineffective esophageal motility (N = 1), distal esophageal spasms (N = 2), and achalasia (N = 7). According to the previously mentioned impedance criteria 21 of 22 swallows with normal barium emptying showed complete transit (96%), and 31 of 32 swallows with severe stasis showed incomplete transit (97%), underscoring that impedance correctly identifies swallows with complete and incomplete bolus transit in different patient groups.

CONVENTIONAL IMPEDANCE MANOMETRY

Early in the development of combined impedance manometry, studies in healthy volunteers were performed in order to establish normal values for this method. In a multicenter study including 60 healthy volunteers, the author and colleagues evaluated bolus transit for liquid and viscous (semisolid) boluses.[5] This allowed defining normal values for bolus presence time at various levels in the esophagus, total bolus transit time for liquids, and viscous swallows (**Table 1**). Using the 90th to 95th percentiles,

Table 1
Normal values for bolus transit assessed using conventional impedance manometry based on data collected in healthy volunteers

Study	N	Bolus Presence Time Distal Esophagus (s)		Bolus Transit Time (s)		Swallows with Complete Bolus Transit (%)	
		Liquid	Viscous	Liquid	Viscous	Liquid	Viscous
Tutuian et al,[5] 2003	60	2.3–9.3	1.5–6.3	5.2–11.9	5.9–12.4	≥80	≥70
Nguyen et al,[8] 2005	42	4.7–9.6	3.4–9.9	5.3–14.9	6.0–17.0	≥80	≥70
Chen et al,[9] 2007	18	5.1–8.1	2.7–5.8	5.9–9.6	7.6–10.7	≥70	≥70
Chen et al,[10] 2013	18		2.4–4.9		6.9–9.9		≥70

it was observed that normal individuals have a complete bolus transit (defined as bolus entrance in the proximal esophagus and bolus exit in all distal esophageal measuring sites) in at least 80% of liquid and in at least 70% of viscous swallows. Conversely, patients with more than 20% of swallows with incomplete bolus transit for liquid and more than 30% of swallows with incomplete bolus transit for viscous are considered to have abnormal bolus transit for liquid and viscous, respectively. These observations were subsequently confirmed by European[8] and Asian[9,10] studies in healthy individuals.

Using the established normal values, the authors reported on the results of esophageal function testing in a group of 350 patients presenting with various esophageal symptoms and having various manometric findings.[11] In this group of patients, the authors found abnormal bolus transit in all patients with achalasia and scleroderma, proving the principle that impedance can assess bolus transit in patients with severe esophageal motility abnormalities. On the other hand, almost all (ie, 95% or more) patients with normal esophageal manometry, nutcracker esophagus, and isolated LES abnormalities (ie, hypertensive, hypotensive, and poorly relaxing LES) had normal bolus transit for liquid. In the group of patients with ineffective esophageal motility (IEM) and distal esophageal spasm (DES), it was noticed that approximately half of the patients had normal bolus transit.

Conchillo and colleagues[12] reported on data from 40 consecutive patients with non-obstructive dysphagia (NOD) investigated using combined impedance manometry. Manometric findings were normal motility in 20 patients; IEM was found in 13 patients. DES was found in 4 patients, and achalasia was found in 3 patients. Normal bolus transit (defined as ≥80% of liquid and ≥70% of viscous swallows with complete bolus transit) was noted in 64.7% patients with normal manometry, in 34.3% of patients with DES, in 23.1% of patients with IEM, and in no (0%) patients with achalasia. Based on these findings, the authors concluded that combined impedance manometry can be used to identify esophageal function abnormalities in NOD patients with normal manometry, IEM, and DES.

Cho and colleagues[13] presented results in 89 subjects including 26 healthy volunteers (62 women, 27 man) who underwent esophageal function testing using combined MII-EM measurements. In this group, 50 (56%) patients had normal esophageal manometry; 17 (19%) patients had IEM, and 7 (8%) patients had nutcracker esophagus. Eleven (12%) patients had scleroderma esophagus, and 4 (5%) patients had achalasia. During liquid swallows, patients with normal manometry had 88 plus or minus 18% swallows with complete bolus transit; patients with IEM had 59 plus or minus 16% swallows with complete bolus transit. Patients with nutcracker esophagus had 98 plus or minus 8% swallows with complete bolus transit. In contrast, patients with scleroderma and achalasia had 9 plus or minus 14% and 5 plus or minus 10% swallows with complete bolus transit, respectively. Normal bolus transit (ie, ≥80% of liquid swallows with complete bolus transit) was noted in all patients with nutcracker esophagus (100%), 80% patients with normal manometry, 54% of patients with IEM, and none (0%) of the patients with scleroderma and achalasia.

A study in 70 patients with IEM identified that there is no perfect (ie, highly sensitive and highly specific) manometric cut-off that would predict complete bolus transit and that the current manometric criteria for diagnosing IEM (ie, 30% or more manometric ineffective swallows) is too sensitive and lacks the specificity of identifying patients with abnormal bolus transit.[14] Normal bolus transit in the group of patients with IEM appeared to be dependent on the distal esophageal amplitude (ie, average amplitude at 2 distal esophageal sites 5 and 10 cm above the LES), the number of sites with low contraction amplitudes, and the overall number of manometric ineffective swallows.

Another important finding of this study was that approximately one-third of patients with IEM had normal bolus transit for liquid and viscous boluses (suggesting a mild functional defect); approximately one-third had abnormal bolus transit for either liquid or viscous boluses (ie, moderate functional defect), and the remaining one-third of IEM patients had abnormal bolus transit for both liquid and viscous boluses (ie, severe functional defect).

A similar analysis in 71 patients with DES indicated that approximately half of patients with manometric criteria of DES have normal bolus transit for both liquid and viscous swallows (ie, no functional defect). About 25% of DES patients had abnormal bolus transit for both liquid and viscous boluses (ie, severe functional defect), and the other 25% had abnormal bolus transit for either liquid or viscous boluses (ie, moderate functional defect).[15] The author and colleagues also noticed manometric and bolus transit differences in DES patients presenting with chest pain and patients presenting primarily with dysphagia. Patients presenting primarily with chest pain had higher contraction amplitudes and a higher proportion of swallows with normal bolus transit time when compared with patients presenting primarily with dysphagia. Based on these observations, one can speculate that DES patients with chest pain, higher amplitude contractions, and normal transit should be managed differently than DES patients with dysphagia, lower amplitude contractions, and abnormal transit.

The importance of assessing bolus transit has been highlighted by study in 80 consecutive patients who underwent laparoscopic fundoplication.[16] These patients were separated into 4 groups based on the presence or absence of symptoms (ie, dysphagia) and normal or abnormal anatomy: group 1 dysphagia and normal anatomy, group 2 dysphagia and abnormal anatomy, group 3 no dysphagia and abnormal anatomy, and group 4 no dysphagia and normal anatomy. The authors found that patients with dysphagia (groups 1 and 2) had similar peristalsis (manometry), but were more likely to have impaired clearance by MII than those without dysphagia (62% vs 32%, $P = .01$), and patients with abnormal anatomy (groups 2 and 3) were also more likely to have impaired esophageal clearance (66% vs 38%, $P = .01$). Finally, of patients who had normal fundoplication anatomy, those with dysphagia were much more likely to have impaired clearance than those with dysphagia (52% vs 21%, $P = .03$). Based on these findings, the authors concluded that most patients with postoperative dysphagia have impaired clearance, even if they have normal fundoplication anatomy and normal peristalsis. Furthermore, impedance measurements may better refine disorders in esophageal motility than conventional manometry alone.

In summary, current data support that combined impedance and manometry can be used in research and clinical settings, providing more detailed information on esophageal function testing compared with conventional manometry alone.

HIGH-RESOLUTION IMPEDANCE MANOMETRY

In the first years, HRM/EPT and combined MII-EM were developed in competition with each other until technical and software development allowed device companies to offer combined high-resolution impedance manometry (HRiM) systems. The combined HRiM provides a unique tool that has the ability to evaluate pressure changes from the hypopharynx to the proximal stomach and determine the efficiency of esophageal peristalsis to propel boluses through the esophagus.

Isocontour pressure topography has become the standard in displaying high-resolution manometry data. Spectral or custom-set color palettes are used to display

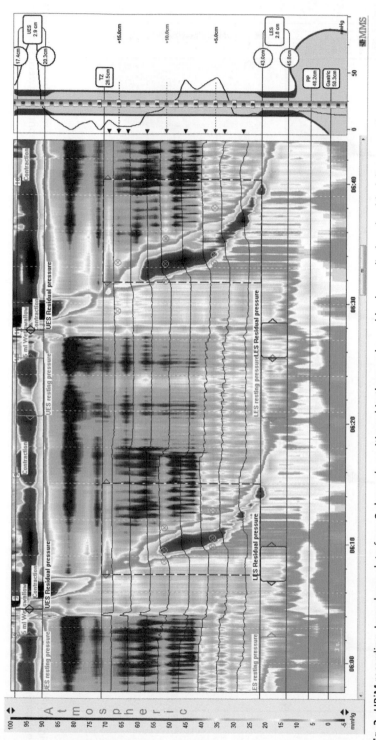

Fig. 3. HRiM recording. Impedance data from 8 channels positioned in the esophageal body are displayed as black lines over the pressure topography plots of HRM. This example shows a normal swallow with complete bolus clearance followed by a spontaneous reflux episode out of the hiatal hernia, followed by another normal swallow clearing the esophageal content.

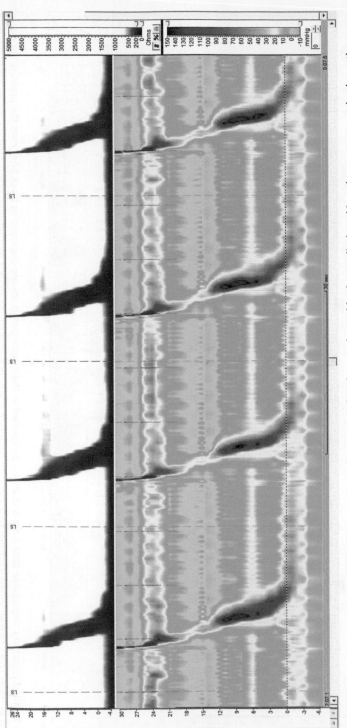

Fig. 4. HRiM recording. Impedance data from 16 channels positioned in the esophageal body are displayed in color-contour mode above the pressure topography plots of HRM. This example shows 4 normal swallows with complete bolus transit (ie, impedance returns to normal between swallows).

pressure gradients, cold colors (blue-green) being attributed to low pressures, and warm colors (yellow-orange-red) being used to indicate high pressures. Displaying the impedance data can be done by overlaying data from individual impedance-measuring segments on the pressure topography colors (**Fig. 3**) using a single-color gradient (ie, gray or purple) to overlay impedance on pressure data or using split screens to display pressure topography and impedance topography on the same time axis (**Fig. 4**). The time synchronization is key to assessing the effect of contraction on bolus transit. For optimal display, the pressure and/or impedance color assignment scale needs to be adjusted; thus pictorial representations should always been displayed with the corresponding scales.

With regards to the analysis of HRiM data, novel approaches have been proposed. These incorporate the definitions of the Chicago classification system of swallows and motility abnormalties,[17] together with a set of pressure and impedance parameters (**Table 2**) that allow an automated impedance manometry evaluation of swallows.[18] According to a recent study, the automated impedance manometry (AIM) parameters have a very high intra- and inter-rater agreement with intra-class correlation coefficients of 0.96 and 0.91 for liquid and viscous swallows, respectively. First, studies in patients with nonobstructive dysphagia (NOD) and normal esophageal manometry indicate that AIM parameters and analysis are superior to the conventional impedance analysis algorithm in providing more plausible explanations for dysphagia than conventional impedance parameters (95% vs 18%; $P<.01$).[19]

Using the AIM parameters, Myers and colleagues[20] analyzed pre- and postfundoplication HRiM recordings in patients undergoing Nissen fundoplication. Of the 19 patients who underwent HRiM testing before and after surgery, 15 developed some dysphagia, including 7 patients with new-onset dysphagia. Using time from nadir esophageal impedance to peak esophageal pressure (TNadImp-PeakP), median intrabolus pressure (IBP, mm Hg), and the rate of bolus pressure rise (IBP slope, mm Hg(-1)) the authors

Table 2	
Definition of variables used by the automated impedance manometry (AIM) analysis	
Variable	**Description of Variable**
Peak pressure (mm Hg)	Mean peak pressure of the esophageal peristalsis
Pressure at nadir impedance (mm Hg)	Mean pressure at the nadir impedance for the bolus
Intrabolus pressure (mm Hg)	Mean intrabolus pressure, defined as the median pressure at the midpoint from the time of nadir impedance to peak pressure
20 mm Hg isocontour defect (cm)	Axial length of the break in peristaltic wave where the peak pressure does not reach 20 mm Hg
Intrabolus pressure slope (mm Hg/s)	Change in pressure over time, from pressure at nadir impedance to pressure at midpoint of time from nadir impedance to peak pressure
Time from nadir impedance to peak pressure (s)	Time interval between nadir esophageal impedance and peak esophageal pressure of peristalsis
Impedance at peak pressure (Ω)	Mean impedance at the peak pressure of the esophageal peristalsis
Ratio of nadir impedance and impedance at peak pressure	Ratio of nadir impedance during the liquid bolus compared with mean impedance at the peak pressure of the esophageal peristalsis
Integrated relaxation pressure 4 s (IRP4)	Lowest 4 seconds cumulative relaxation pressure of the esophagogastric junction during a swallow

proposed a dysphagia risk index (DRI = IBP × IBP_slope/TNadImp-PeakP) as an integrated parameter to predict postfundoplication dysphagia. The DRI values in patients with postoperative dysphagia were significantly higher than in those without dysphagia (dysphagia DRI = 58, interquartile range [IQR] = 21–408 vs no dysphagia DRI = 9, IQR = 2–19, $P<.02$). Based on these findings, the authors proposed a DRI greater than 14 as the optimal predictor of postfundoplication dysphagia (sensitivity 75% and specificity 93%). Although these results need further validation, these data suggest that AIM analysis would be able to identify pre-existing subclinical variation of esophageal function that would predict the risk of developing postfundoplication dysphagia.

SUMMARY

Esophageal bolus transit assessed by multichannel intraluminal impedance offers the opportunity to identify and quantify bolus movements through the esophagus in both healthy volunteers and patients with esophageal symptoms, in particular nonobstructive dysphagia. Data from combined impedance manometry offered a first set of information on esophageal bolus transit and/or retention in patients with various esophageal motility abnormalities. The combination of HRiM offers a new tool with several novel parameters that should help find better explanations for esophageal symptoms.

REFERENCES

1. Silny J. Intraluminal multiple electric impedance procedure for measurement of gastrointestinal motility. J Gastrointest Motil 1991;3:151–62. Available at: http://onlinelibrary.wiley.com/doi/10.1111/j.1365-2982.1991.tb00061.x/abstract.
2. Blom D, Mason RJ, Balaji NS, et al. Esophageal bolus transport identified by simultaneous multichannel intraluminal impedance and manofluoroscopy [abstract]. Gastroenterology 2001;120:P103.
3. Srinivasan R, Vela MF, Katz PO, et al. Esophageal function testing using multichannel intraluminal impedance. Am J Physiol Gastrointest Liver Physiol 2001; 280:G457–62.
4. Simren M, Silny J, Holloway R, et al. Relevance of ineffective oesophageal motility during oesophageal acid clearance. Gut 2003;52:784–90.
5. Tutuian R, Vela MF, Balaji NS, et al. Esophageal function testing with combined multichannel intraluminal impedance and manometry: multicenter study in healthy volunteers. Clin Gastroenterol Hepatol 2003;1:174–82.
6. Imam H, Shay S, Ali A, et al. Bolus transit patterns in healthy subjects: a study using simultaneous impedance monitoring, videoesophagram, and esophageal manometry. Am J Physiol Gastrointest Liver Physiol 2005;288:G1000–6.
7. Cho YK, Choi MG, Oh SN, et al. Comparison of bolus transit patterns identified by esophageal impedance to barium esophagram in patients with dysphagia. Dis Esophagus 2012;25:17–25.
8. Nguyen NQ, Rigda R, Tippett M, et al. Assessment of oesophageal motor function using combined perfusion manometry and multi-channel intra-luminal impedance measurement in normal subjects. Neurogastroenterol Motil 2005;17:458–65.
9. Chen CL, Yi CH. Assessment of esophageal motor function using combined multichannel intraluminal impedance and manometry in healthy volunteers: a single-center study in Taiwan. J Gastroenterol Hepatol 2007;22:1039–43.
10. Chen CL, Yi CH, Chou AS, et al. Esophageal solid bolus transit: studies using combined multichannel intraluminal impedance and manometry in healthy volunteers. Dis Esophagus 2013;26:91–6.

11. Tutuian R, Castell DO. Combined multichannel intraluminal impedance and manometry clarifies esophageal function abnormalities. Study in 350 patients. Am J Gastroenterol 2004;99:1011–9.
12. Conchillo JM, Nguyen NQ, Samsom M, et al. Multichannel intraluminal impedance monitoring in the evaluation of patients with non-obstructive dysphagia. Am J Gastroenterol 2005;100:2624–32.
13. Cho YK, Choi MG, Park JM, et al. Evaluation of esophageal function in patients with esophageal motor abnormalities using multichannel intraluminal impedance esophageal manometry. World J Gastroenterol 2006;12:6349–54.
14. Tutuian R, Castell DO. Clarification of the esophageal function defect in patients with manometric ineffective esophageal motility: studies using combined impedance-manometry. Clin Gastroenterol Hepatol 2004;2:230–6.
15. Tutuian R, Mainie I, Agrawal A, et al. Symptom and function heterogenicity among patients with distal esophageal spasm. Studies using combined impedance-manometry. Am J Gastroenterol 2006;101:464–9.
16. Yigit T, Quiroga E, Oelschlager B. Multichannel intraluminal impedance for the assessment of post-fundoplication dysphagia. Dis Esophagus 2006;19:382–8.
17. Bredenoord AJ, Fox M, Kahrilas PJ, et al. Chicago classification criteria of esophageal motility disorders defined in high-resolution esophageal pressure topography. Neurogastroenterol Motil 2012;24(Suppl 1):57–65.
18. Rohof WO, Myers JC, Estremera FA, et al. Inter- and intra-rater reproducibility of automated and integrated pressure-flow analysis of esophageal pressure-impedance recordings. Neurogastroenterol Motil 2014;26:168–75.
19. Nguyen NQ, Holloway RH, Smout AJ, et al. Automated impedance-manometry analysis detects esophageal motor dysfunction in patients who have non-obstructive dysphagia with normal manometry. Neurogastroenterol Motil 2013; 25:238–45.
20. Myers JC, Nguyen NQ, Jamieson GG, et al. Susceptibility to dysphagia after fundoplication revealed by novel automated impedance manometry analysis. Neurogastroenterol Motil 2012;24:812.e393.

Measuring Mechanical Properties of the Esophageal Wall Using Impedance Planimetry

An Moonen, MD, Guy Boeckxstaens, MD, PhD*

KEYWORDS

- Impedance planimetry • FLIP • Distensibility • Esophagus
- Esophagogastric junction

KEY POINTS

- Impedance planimetry allows accurate measurement of compliance or distensibility.
- Distensibility is a better parameter than pressure alone to evaluate sphincter competence.
- Distensibility of the esophagogastric junction (EGJ) is increased in gastroesophageal reflux disease patients and normalized by fundoplication.
- Untreated achalasia patients have a lower distensibility of the EGJ than well-treated achalasia patients and healthy volunteers.
- In achalasia, EGJ distensibility correlates with symptom severity and may therefore play a potentially important role in the clinical management of achalasia.
- Functional lumen imaging probe technology may provide valuable perioperative information on EGJ distensibility during Heller myotomy, peroral endoscopic myotomy, and anti-reflux surgery.

INTRODUCTION

The esophagus is a muscular tube, serving as a conduit between the oral cavity and the stomach with its principle role to transport ingested material toward the stomach. At its distal end, the lower esophageal sphincter (LES) is continuously contracted to

Funding Sources: G. Boeckxstaens is supported by a grant (Odysseus Program, G.0905.07) of the Flemish 'Fonds Wetenschappelijk Onderzoek' (FWO). A. Moonen is performing a doctoral fellowship, supported by the Flemisch 'Fonds Wetenschappelijk Onderzoek' (FWO).
Conflict of Interest: There are no conflicts of interest.
Department of Gastroenterology, Translational Research Center for Gastrointestinal Disorders (TARGID), University Hospital of Leuven, Catholic University of Leuven, Herestraat 49, Leuven 3000, Belgium
* Corresponding author.
E-mail address: Guy.Boeckxstaens@med.kuleuven.be

http://dx.doi.org/10.1016/j.giec.2014.06.001
1052-5157/14/$ – see front matter © 2014 Elsevier Inc. All rights reserved.

prevent reflux of gastric contents. Sphincter competence and more specific competence of the esophagogastric junction (EGJ) involve a complex interaction between LES tone, diaphragmatic contraction during the respiratory cycle, and the valvular effect caused by the sling fibers. More than 40 years ago, Harris and Pope[1] identified that resistance to distension by measurement of radial force rather than sphincter pressure should be the prime determinant of sphincteric strength. Hence, measuring pressure and cross-sectional areas (CSA) of the EGJ would be a better parameter to evaluate sphincter competence. Conversely, transport of intraluminal contents across the EGJ is largely determined by the diameter of the EGJ.[2] Pandolfino and colleagues[2] indeed elegantly demonstrated that volume flow across the EGJ can be estimated by using a simplified mathematical model based on Newton's law of motion. From this model, it is evident that flow is highly dependent on the diameter of the EGJ, given that it is factored to the 4th power in the equation of the mathematical model. Based on these findings, it is becoming increasingly clear that not basal pressure generated by the EGJ but rather its ability to open or distend is the main determinant of flow, in either antegrade or retrograde direction. Hence, clinical tools measuring distensibility may prove to be more useful to assess the function of the EGJ.

EARLIER METHODS TO MEASURE DISTENSIBILITY

In 2002, Pandolfino and colleagues[2] elegantly combined distension of the EGJ using a barostat balloon with barium swallow images to assess the EGJ distensibility. The balloon pressure was set at 5 mm Hg and was subsequently increased in 2-mm Hg increments until opening of the EGJ was noted fluoroscopically. In addition, the diameter of the EGJ was assessed during 5-mL dilute barium swallows at different barostat balloon pressures. Distensibility was then defined as the relationship between the EGJ diameter (measured by barium swallow) and balloon distension pressure. This technique was performed in 8 healthy volunteers and 9 reflux patients with a hiatal hernia. The distensibility of the EGJ was significantly increased in gastroesophageal reflux disease (GERD) patients with a hiatus hernia such that the opening occurred at a significantly lower distension pressure and that for a given distension pressure the resultant opening diameter was on average 0.5 cm wider.

The underlying hypothesis for measuring the compliance of the EGJ during LES relaxation was that the observed increased diameters in hernia patients would both qualitatively and quantitatively determine retrograde gastroesophageal flow. Using a mathematical model based on Newton's law of motion, it is indeed evident that flow is highly dependent on diameter, given that it is factored to the 4th power. Furthermore, using this model together with the pressure and diameter measurements described above, estimations for esophagogastric flow across the EGJ for water and air were made for healthy volunteers as well as GERD patients with a hiatal hernia. The flow for either air or water was 2-fold to 3-fold greater for the hernia group compared with normal subjects at each value of gastroesophageal pressure gradient. Within each group, flow of air is about 2 orders of magnitude greater than the flow of water. Thus, the lower opening pressure and 0.5-cm increase in EGJ diameter observed in hernia patients coupled with the difference in viscosity between water and air make a normal individual capable of venting large volumes of gas from the stomach at low pressure with minimal potential for liquid reflux, whereas hernia patients will vent large volumes of air or water at similar pressures. A correlate of this is that the volume of refluxate is also uniformly higher among hernia patients. Taken together, this study of Pandolfino[2] showed that measuring opening patterns and distensibility can be an indicator of the status of the junction in health or disease.

However, this early method using barostat and fluoroscopy is cumbersome because it involves radiation and therefore is not suitable for clinical practice.

PRINCIPLE OF IMPEDANCE PLANIMETRY

In 1971, Harris and colleagues[3] described a method to assess the CSA of the ureter using impedance measurements between 4 different electrodes placed on a thin probe. It took another 10 years, however, before Colstrup and colleagues[4] developed an expandable nonconductible balloon containing electrodes, allowing the measurement of biomechanical wall properties. This technique is based on the principle that the CSA is inversely proportional to the voltage across the sensing electrodes if a current passes through a polyurethane bag filled with saline. If all other parameters are kept constant, the impedance is proportional to the CSA of the bag between the sensing electrodes (**Fig. 1**).

In contrast to the barostat, whereby distension data are based on pressure-volume relationships, impedance planimetry enables actual measurement of CSA during balloon distension, which correlates better to diametrical changes in the digestive lumen.[5] Although several studies have validated the use of impedance planimetry in the esophagus of healthy volunteers and patients,[6] few studies have been performed in sphincter regions due to several technical limitations. First, accurate positioning of the electrode in the sphincteric region is rather difficult. Second, there is a tendency for bag displacement during distension in a high pressure zone such as a sphincter. To overcome this, a multielectrode probe has been created allowing the simultaneous recording of CSA at different positions.[7] McMahon and colleagues[7] proved that this multielectrode technique is indeed capable of generating an illustration of the geometric changes in the EGJ, thereby profiling the lumen of the organ under study. This probe is known as the functional lumen imaging probe (FLIP), which has recently become commercially available (endoFLIP; Crospon Medical Divices, Galway, Ireland). It consists of a 240-cm-long catheter with a 14-cm bag, compliant to a maximal diameter of 25 mm, attached to its distal end. Inside the bag, 17 electrodes are placed at 4-mm intervals. An excitation current of 100 μA is generated between 2 adjacent electrodes at a frequency of 5 kHz. Using impedance planimetry, CSAs are

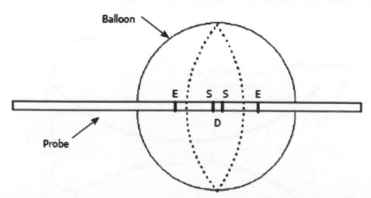

Fig. 1. Schematic representation of a conventional impedance planimeter probe with a single set of exiting (E) and sensing (S) electrodes for the measurement of CSA in the middle of the bag. D, distance between the sensing electrodes. (*From* McMahon BP, Drewes AM, Gregersen H. Functional oesophago-gastric junction imaging. World J Gastroenterol 2006;12(18):2818–24; with permission.)

determined for the 16 cross-sections during volume-controlled distensions. In addition, 2 pressure sensors determine intrabag pressure, allowing assessment of EGJ distensibility (**Fig. 2**).

FUNCTIONAL LUMINAL IMAGING AND EGJ DISEASE
Healthy Volunteers

It is clear from several studies that FLIP measurement can be performed easily and safely. It can be performed during endoscopy or as a separate procedure; in either case, the FLIP probe is mostly well tolerated. Kwiatek and colleagues[8] performed a study in 20 healthy volunteers. The FLIP procedure was performed during a routine esophagogastroduodenoscopy, where the FLIP probe was passed through the endoscopic instrumentation channel and positioned across the EGJ. All patients received moderate sedation during the procedure (5–15 mg midazolam, 20–200 µg fentanyl). In healthy volunteers, a mean CSA of 94 (27–225) mm^2 was measured at the 30 mL distension of the FLIP bag and a mean CSA of 264 (99–496) mm^2 was seen at the 40 mL distension, corresponding with an intrabag pressure of 25 (6–47) and 39 (17–60) mm Hg, respectively. EGJ distensibility (CSA vs pressure) was based on the narrowest CSA and the corresponding intrabag pressure and expressed as the EGJ distensibility index (DI) at each distention volume. The index was calculated as [narrowest CSA/(intrabag pressure + intragastric pressure offset)], wherein intragastric pressure was given as 4.0 mm Hg based on previous reports of typical normal intragastric pressure values across healthy controls. The DI was 4 (1–14) mm^2/mm Hg at the 30 mL distension and 6 (4–8) mm^2/mm Hg at the 40 mL distension.

The study of Rohof and colleagues[9] confirmed these results. In this study, 15 healthy volunteers were studied. The FLIP procedure was performed as a separate procedure, without sedation. Healthy volunteers had a mean EGJ distensibility of 6.3 ± 0.7 mm^2/mm Hg using a 50-mL volume distension.

GERD

GERD is one of the most common digestive diseases in the Western world, resulting from repetitive exposure of the esophagus to gastric contents. Given the high prevalence of GERD, understanding of the pathophysiology is of great importance. In the following section, the evidence indicating that increased EGJ compliance is one of

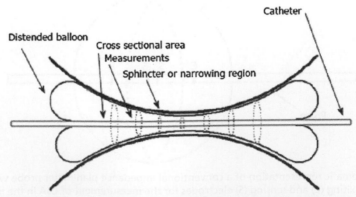

Fig. 2. Schematic view of the FLIP probe distended in the region of the esophagogastric junction. (*From* McMahon BP, Drewes AM, Gregersen H. Functional oesophago-gastric junction imaging. World J Gastroenterol 2006;12(18):2818–24; with permission.)

the pathophysiological abnormalities contributing to increased esophageal acid exposure is reviewed.

Functional measurement

Currently, EGJ distensibility measurement is mostly performed using a commercially developed device (ie, the EndoFLIP). This probe consists of a 240-cm-long catheter with a 14-cm balloon attached to its distal end positioned in the esophagus with the impedance electrodes straddling the EGJ at the center of the balloon. In most distension protocols, the balloon is inflated to a 20-mL, 30-mL, 40-mL, and 50-mL volume. Pressures and CSAs are collected at a rate of 10 Hz. Distensibility is assessed using the median value over a 30-second dynamic measurement of the narrowest CSA, which corresponds to the EGJ, and the median intrabag pressure.

Kwiatek and colleagues[8] measured EGJ distensibility in 20 healthy volunteers and 20 GERD patients without hiatal hernia. In both groups, the least distensible locus at the EGJ was usually at the hiatus. As a group, GERD patients exhibited 2-fold to 3-fold increased EGJ distensibility compared with controls, particularly at 20-mL to 30-mL distention volumes. These values are quantitatively similar to the previous measurements using barostat balloon distension of the EGJ.[2] However, these findings could not be confirmed in the study of Tucker and colleagues.[10] In this study, 22 healthy volunteers and 18 GERD patients were included, surprisingly showing that patients with reflux symptoms had a lower CSA and distensibility than healthy volunteers. A possible explanation for this controversy could be the difference in control group used, given that 14% of the healthy volunteers had a pathologic acid exposure on wireless pH monitoring.

As an increased distensibility is part of the underlying pathophysiological abnormalities in GERD, efficient treatment should aim to correct this abnormality. Indeed, Blom and colleagues[11] showed a significant reduction of distensibility after antireflux surgery. Distensibility was determined in 15 patients who underwent Nissen fundoplication using custom-made catheter before and after surgery with the patient under general anesthesia. These results are in line with the earlier barostat study of Pandolfino.[12] In this study, EGJ opening pressure and opening diameter after fundoplication were decreased to levels similar to normal subjects.

Intraoperative measurement

Laparoscopic Nissen fundoplication is the surgical treatment of choice for GERD. However, this procedure may be associated with complications, such as dysphagia, gas bloat, and inability to belch and vomit, as a result of a too-tight fundic wrap. Therefore, intraoperative measurement of distensibility could possibly guide the surgeon to determine the optimal size of the fundic wrap, thereby preventing or reducing the risk of these postoperative complications. Ilczyszyn and Botha[13] studied the feasibility of intraoperative distensibility measurement using the FLIP probe. Intraoperative FLIP measurement was performed in 17 subjects without perioperative and postoperative complications. Hiatus repair and fundoplication result in a significant overall reduction in the median distensibility at 30-mL and 40-mL distensions (30-mL balloon distension reduction of 3.26 mm^2/mm Hg [$P = .0087$], 40 mL balloon distension reduction of 2.39 mm^2/mm Hg [$P = .0039$]). Of interest, intraoperative distensibility was very low (0.47 mm^2/mm Hg) in one patient, who subsequently required reoperation because of significant symptoms of dysphagia. Another patient in the series had a fundoplication that appeared visually too tight. FLIP measurement showed a low DI of 0.65 mm^2/mm Hg. Based on this FLIP measurement, the procedure was converted intraoperatively to a Lind 270° wrap, resulting in a change in the DI from 0.65 to

0.89 mm²/mm Hg. Afterward, this patient had no symptoms of dysphagia. These data elegantly show that the EndoFLIP system could be useful to help the surgeon construct the optimal fundic wrap. Further studies are needed to confirm improved clinical results and reduction of postoperative dysphagia or gas bloat following antireflux surgery when combined with intraoperative assessment of EGJ distensibility.

Achalasia

Achalasia is the best characterized esophageal motility disorder. It is caused by disappearance of inhibitory neurons leading to a loss of peristalsis and defective relaxation of the LES. The subsequent retention of food in the esophagus results in the typical symptoms of achalasia (ie, dysphagia, regurgitation of undigested food, chest pain, and weight loss). As the neuronal loss is irreversible, there is no curative treatment of achalasia. Although the pathophysiology of achalasia is associated with impairment of both peristalsis and LES relaxation, treatment is focused on reducing EGJ pressure to improve bolus passage and thereby ameliorating symptoms. Recent insight, however, revealed that not only basal sphincter pressure but also distensibility of the EGJ is a major determinant of esophageal emptying and thus therapeutic success. Indeed, Rohof and colleagues[9] showed that compliance was significantly reduced in untreated achalasia patients and patients with recurrent symptoms compared with controls and that distensibility was increased after treatment. Moreover, in patients with achalasia, EGJ distensibility correlates with esophageal emptying and symptoms. Therefore, impedance planimetry can be of use in the management of achalasia.

Intraoperative measurement

Current treatment modalities to lower LES tone consist of pneumatic dilation, laparoscopic Heller myotomy (LHM), and peroral endoscopic myotomy (POEM). Surgical treatment of achalasia involves myotomy of the LES; however, it remains difficult for the surgeon to estimate the completeness of the myotomy. The same applies to the most recently introduced treatment of achalasia (ie, POEM). During POEM, a submucosal tunnel is created during endoscopy to reach the LES and to dissect the circular muscle fibers over a 7- to 10-cm esophageal and 2-cm gastric length.

As the completeness of the myotomy is not always easy to assess, some investigators have tried to improve surgical success rates by measuring the residual LES pressure using perioperative manometry.[14] Of interest, manometry could indeed identify persistent high pressure zone, suggestive of incomplete myotomy, that could be corrected during surgery with further section of circular muscle fibers.[14,15]

In line, endoFLIP has been used as an adjunctive guide during Heller myotomy or POEM. Teitelbaum and colleagues[16] recently published the results of perioperative distensibility changes measured by FLIP in 29 patients who underwent LHM or POEM. FLIP could be performed intraoperatively in 86% of patients showing a significant increase in CSA at 40-mL FLIP distension after myotomy in LHM and POEM. In addition, intrabag pressure decreased significantly after POEM (mean pre 34 ± 9.5 mm Hg vs mean post 21.8 ± 6.2 mm Hg; P<.001), whereas LHM resulted only in a trend toward decreased intrabag pressure at a 40-mL distension volume (mean pre 32.4 ± 14.1 mm Hg vs mean post 25 ± 9.5 mm Hg; P = .08). The DI increased significantly following LHM (mean pre 1.4 ± 1.3 mm²/mm Hg vs mean post 7.6 ± 4.4 mm²/mm Hg; P<.001). POEM led to a similar increase (mean pre 1.4 ± 1.9 mm²/mm Hg vs mean post 7.9 ± 2.7 mm²/mm Hg; P<.001).

These data illustrate that intraoperative recording of distensibility is feasible with FLIP and that both LHM and POEM result in a comparable 4-fold to 5-fold increase in distensibility. Most interestingly, these studies show that intraoperative FLIP has the potential to be used during LHM and POEM to calibrate the myotomy and fundoplication, and to ensure an adequate release of the EGJ.

Functional measurement

With regard to the clinical management of achalasia, it is important to identify patients in need of re-treatment to prevent long-term complications, such as dilatation of the esophagus and increased risk to develop dysplasia. Identification of these patients is often challenging because symptoms do not correlate with functional parameters, mainly because patients get used to symptoms and adapt their diet accordingly. Therefore, objective functional markers evaluating the EGJ are needed. Several studies have proposed manometry to be a useful test to determine whether patients should be re-treated. In general, LES pressure lower than 10 mm Hg after therapy has been reported to be a good predictor of treatment success.[17–19] However, other studies and clinical experience contradict these results, especially because a significant proportion of patients have persistent symptoms despite low LES pressure.[9,20–22] Interestingly, these patients have incomplete esophageal emptying on a timed barium esophagogram,[21,23] while a significant proportion of these patients benefit from additional treatment with pneumodilation. These observations argue against LES pressure as a useful test to assess the need for treatment. Recent findings suggest that assessment of distensibility may represent a better approach to identify patients in need of re-treatment. FLIP data indeed correlated better with esophageal emptying and clinical response compared with manometry (**Fig. 3**).[9,24] Rohof and colleagues[9] showed that EGJ distensibility was significantly reduced in untreated patients with achalasia, compared with controls (0.7 ± 0.9 mm^2/mm Hg vs 6.3 ± 0.7 mm^2/mm Hg; $P<.001$) and that EGJ distensibility correlated with esophageal emptying ($r = -0.72$; $P<.01$) and symptoms ($r = 0.61$; $P<.01$). Moreover, distensibility was significantly increased with treatment and was significantly higher in patients successfully treated (Eckardt score <3) compared with those having persistent symptoms (1.6 ± 0.3 vs 4.4 ± 0.5 mm^2/mm Hg, respectively, $P = .001$). Furthermore, a cutoff value for treatment success and failure was determined. A value of less than 2.9 mm^2/mm Hg at the 50-mL distension indicated treatment failure with a sensitivity of 92% and a specificity of 72% (**Fig. 4**). Pandolfino and colleagues[24] confirmed these findings in 20 healthy volunteers and 54 achalasia patients. The esophagogastric junction-distensibility index (EGJ-DI) was greatest in control subjects and least in the untreated patients; patients with a good treatment response had significantly greater EGJ-DI than untreated patients or patients with a poor treatment response.

Taken together, these data show that FLIP provides a useful tool to measure EGJ distensibility in achalasia patients. Most importantly, EGJ distensibility correlates with symptom severity and provides complementary information to existing tests, suggesting that this technique may play a potentially important role in the clinical management of achalasia (see **Fig. 3**).

Therapeutic use of impedance planimetry

Pneumodilation is a standard treatment of achalasia. In this treatment, a balloon is expanded in the EGJ to disrupt and widen the LES to improve bolus passage. Pneumodilation is often combined with fluoroscopy to visualize the shape of the balloon and, most importantly, to observe the disappearance of the waist in the balloon during dilation. As impedance planimetry can image the shape and size of the EGJ and esophageal body, it may also be used to replace fluoroscopy during pneumodilation. Against this background, a new device has been developed (EsoFLIP; Crospon) consisting of a noncompliant balloon, suited for pneumodilation, mounted on the FLIP

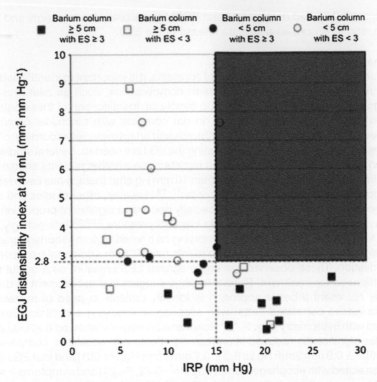

Fig. 3. The relationship between integrated relaxation pressure (IRP), EGJ-DI, bolus retention on timed barium esophagram, and Eckardt score (ES) in the group of treated achalasia patients. The EGJ-DI at 40 mL and IRP are plotted on the axes and the data point for each individual is further characterized based on the ES and barium column height at 5 min. There was a logical concordance between IRP and EGJ-DI at 40 mL in that there was no instance where the 2 were contradictory; there were no instances in which the IRP was abnormal and the EGJ-DI at 40 mL was normal (*dark gray box*). However, there were instances where IRP was normal and patients continued to have either bolus retention or an ES greater than or equal to 3. The cutoff value based on the 95th percentile for EGJ-DI at 40 mL (2.8 mm²/mm Hg) had good discrimination for symptoms. Patients with an EGJ-DI at 40 mL greater than 2.8 mm²/mm Hg and abnormal bolus retention had poor bolus clearance that was not directly related to an obstruction at the EGJ. Reduced emptying in this scenario was associated with low esophageal pressure that may be related to some esophageal dilatation and poor longitudinal muscle function. These defects would prevent the esophagus from pressurizing to a degree that facilitated bolus transit across the EGJ. (*From* Pandolfino JE, de RA, Nicodeme F, et al. Distensibility of the esophagogastric junction assessed with the functional lumen imaging probe (FLIP) in achalasia patients. Neurogastroenterol Motil 2013;25(6):496–501; with permission.)

catheter. Although the first achalasia patient has already been treated with this device, validation against the standard balloon is absolutely required.[25]

FUNCTIONAL LUMINAL IMAGING AND ESOPHAGEAL BODY DISEASE
Eosinophilic Esophagitis

Eosinophilic esophagitis (EoE) is a chronic inflammatory disease of the esophagus, characterized by eosinophilic infiltration of the esophagus, clinically leading to

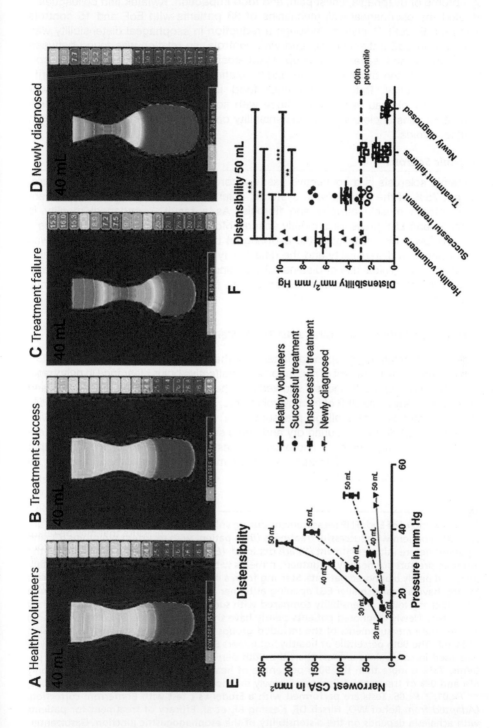

symptoms of dysphagia, chest pain, and food impaction. Kwiatek and colleagues[26] studied the esophageal wall mechanics of 33 patients with EoE and 15 controls using the EndoFLIP system. Although a reduction in esophageal distensibility was observed in EoE patients compared with controls, no relation was found between distensibility and severity of esophageal eosinophilia.[26,27] Nicodème and colleagues,[27] on the other hand, did find a relationship between symptom severity and distensibility. Patients with prior food impaction had significantly lower distensibility plateau values than those with solid food dysphagia only. Up until now, it remains unclear whether distensibility can be restored after treatment with corticosteroids.

Systemic Sclerosis

Systemic sclerosis is a connective tissue disorder involving the skin and viscera. Almost 75% of the patients with systemic sclerosis have esophageal involvement with smooth muscle atrophy and fibrosis. As a result, esophageal motility is impaired and LES pressure is mostly absent. Moreover, Villadsen and colleagues[28] showed lower distensibility of the esophageal body; however, no correlation was found between distensibility and the different types of systemic sclerosis. The implications and clinical use of distensibility testing of the esophagus in scleroderma remain therefore rather limited, especially as no effective treatment is currently available.

FUNCTIONAL LUMINAL IMAGING AND THE UPPER ESOPHAGEAL SPHINCTER

A better understanding of opening patterns of the upper esophageal sphincter (UES) could improve the treatment of aspiration and ineffective bolus clearance in dysphagia patients. Regan and colleagues[29] showed that the FLIP balloon could be inserted and distended safely in the UES of healthy volunteers, providing information on changes in UES diameter and intraballoon pressure after dry and wet swallows. Moreover, maximum UES diameters during dry and liquid swallowing as measured by FLIP are similar to those measured by fluoroscopy. These preliminary findings suggest that FLIP can provide useful information on UES dynamics; however, more research on this subject is definitely needed.

◄─────────

Fig. 4. Examples of EndoFLIP measurement during volumetric distensions in a healthy volunteer (*A*), a patient with successful treatment (*B*), a patient with recurrent symptoms (*C*), and a patient before initial treatment (*D*) are depicted. (*E*) The EGJ opening plotted against the intrabag pressure for healthy volunteers, patients with successful treatment, treatment failures, and newly diagnosed patients. Starting from a 40-mL volumetric distension, treatment failures have a clearly smaller EGJ opening at higher intrabag pressure, corresponding with a significantly lower distensibility compared with successfully treated patients and healthy volunteers. Newly diagnosed patients clearly have the most impaired EGJ distensibility. (*F*) The separate measurements of the included groups at the maximal volumetric distension of 50 mL. The 90th percentile of healthy volunteers EGJ distensibility is marked. Open symbols used in case values are less than the 90th percentile. Of the successfully treated patients, 78% is more than the 90th percentile of healthy volunteers, in contrast with only 8% and 0% of treatment failures and newly diagnosed patients, respectively. *** $P<.001$; ** $P<.01$; * $P<.05$. Tests are performed with a Student's *t* test with Bonferroni correction. (*Adapted from* Rohof WO, Hirsch DP, Kessing BF, et al. Efficacy of treatment for patients with achalasia depends on the distensibility of the esophagogastric junction. Gastroenterology 2012;143(2):328–35; with permission.)

SUMMARY

Impedance planimetry is a novel technique providing valuable information on the mechanical properties of the esophagus and EGJ based on measurement of CSA and intraluminal pressure. This tool may be of clinical use in guiding the clinical management of achalasia while providing valuable perioperative information on EGJ distensibility during Heller myotomy, POEM, and antireflux surgery. Further studies will ultimately determine its true contribution to improve patient management.

REFERENCES

1. Harris LD, Pope CE. "SQUEEZE" VS. RESISTANCE: an evaluation of the mechanism of sphincter competence. J Clin Invest 1964;43:2272–8.
2. Pandolfino JE, Shi G, Curry J, et al. Esophagogastric junction distensibility: a factor contributing to sphincter incompetence. Am J Physiol Gastrointest Liver Physiol 2002;282(6):G1052–8.
3. Harris JH, Therkelsen EE, Zinner NR. Electrical measurements of ureteral flow. In: Boyarsky S, Tanagho EA, Gottschalk CW, et al, editors. Urodynamics. London: Academic Press. p. 465–72.
4. Colstrup H, Mortensen SO, Kristensen JK. A probe for measurements of related values of cross-sectional area and pressure in the resting female urethra. Urol Res 1983;11(3):139–43.
5. Gregersen H, Gilja OH, Hausken T, et al. Mechanical properties in the human gastric antrum using B-mode ultrasonography and antral distension. Am J Physiol Gastrointest Liver Physiol 2002;283(2):G368–75.
6. Gregersen H, Liao D. New perspectives of studying gastrointestinal muscle function. World J Gastroenterol 2006;12(18):2864–9.
7. McMahon BP, Frokjaer JB, Drewes AM, et al. A new measurement of oesophagogastric junction competence. Neurogastroenterol Motil 2004;16(5):543–6.
8. Kwiatek MA, Pandolfino JE, Hirano I, et al. Esophagogastric junction distensibility assessed with an endoscopic functional luminal imaging probe (EndoFLIP). Gastrointest Endosc 2010;72(2):272–8.
9. Rohof WO, Hirsch DP, Kessing BF, et al. Efficacy of treatment for patients with achalasia depends on the distensibility of the esophagogastric junction. Gastroenterology 2012;143(2):328–35.
10. Tucker E, Sweis R, Anggiansah A, et al. Measurement of esophago-gastric junction cross-sectional area and distensibility by an endolumenal functional lumen imaging probe for the diagnosis of gastro-esophageal reflux disease. Neurogastroenterol Motil 2013;25(11):904–10.
11. Blom D, Bajaj S, Liu J, et al. Laparoscopic Nissen fundoplication decreases gastroesophageal junction distensibility in patients with gastroesophageal reflux disease. J Gastrointest Surg 2005;9(9):1318–25.
12. Pandolfino JE, Curry J, Shi G, et al. Restoration of normal distensive characteristics of the esophagogastric junction after fundoplication. Ann Surg 2005;242(1):43–8.
13. Ilczyszyn A, Botha AJ. Feasibility of esophagogastric junction distensibility measurement during Nissen fundoplication. Dis Esophagus 2013. [Epub ahead of print].
14. Nussbaum MS, Jones MP, Pritts TA, et al. Intraoperative manometry to assess the esophagogastric junction during laparoscopic fundoplication and myotomy. Surg Laparosc Endosc Percutan Tech 2001;11(5):294–300.
15. Endo S, Nakajima K, Nishikawa K, et al. Laparoscopic Heller-Dor surgery for esophageal achalasia: impact of intraoperative real-time manometric feedback on postoperative outcomes. Dig Surg 2009;26(4):342–8.

16. Teitelbaum EN, Boris L, Arafat FO, et al. Comparison of esophagogastric junction distensibility changes during POEM and Heller myotomy using intraoperative FLIP. Surg Endosc 2013;27(12):4547–55.
17. Hulselmans M, Vanuytsel T, Degreef T, et al. Long-term outcome of pneumatic dilation in the treatment of achalasia. Clin Gastroenterol Hepatol 2010;8(1):30–5.
18. Eckardt VF, Aignherr C, Bernhard G. Predictors of outcome in patients with achalasia treated by pneumatic dilation. Gastroenterology 1992;103(6):1732–8.
19. Eckardt VF, Gockel I, Bernhard G. Pneumatic dilation for achalasia: late results of a prospective follow up investigation. Gut 2004;53(5):629–33.
20. Katz PO, Richter JE, Cowan R, et al. Apparent complete lower esophageal sphincter relaxation in achalasia. Gastroenterology 1986;90(4):978–83.
21. Amaravadi R, Levine MS, Rubesin SE, et al. Achalasia with complete relaxation of lower esophageal sphincter: radiographic-manometric correlation. Radiology 2005;235(3):886–91.
22. Mearin F, Malagelada JR. Complete lower esophageal sphincter relaxation observed in some achalasia patients is functionally inadequate. Am J Physiol Gastrointest Liver Physiol 2000;278(3):G376–83.
23. Rohof WO, Lei A, Boeckxstaens GE. Esophageal stasis on a timed barium esophagogram predicts recurrent symptoms in patients with long-standing achalasia. Am J Gastroenterol 2013;108(1):49–55.
24. Pandolfino JE, de RA, Nicodeme F, et al. Distensibility of the esophagogastric junction assessed with the functional lumen imaging probe (FLIP) in achalasia patients. Neurogastroenterol Motil 2013;25(6):496–501.
25. O'Dea J, Siersema PD. Esophageal dilation with integrated balloon imaging: initial evaluation in a porcine model. Therap Adv Gastroenterol 2013;6(2):109–14.
26. Kwiatek MA, Hirano I, Kahrilas PJ, et al. Mechanical properties of the esophagus in eosinophilic esophagitis. Gastroenterology 2011;140(1):82–90.
27. Nicodème F, Hirano I, Chen J, et al. Esophageal distensibility as a measure of disease severity in patients with eosinophilic esophagitis. Clin Gastroenterol Hepatol 2013;11(9):1101–7.
28. Villadsen GE, Storkholm J, Zachariae H, et al. Oesophageal pressure-cross-sectional area distributions and secondary peristalsis in relation to subclassification of systemic sclerosis. Neurogastroenterol Motil 2001;13(3):199–210.
29. Regan J, Walshe M, Rommel N, et al. A new evaluation of the upper esophageal sphincter using the functional lumen imaging probe: a preliminary report. Dis Esophagus 2013;26(2):117–23.

Evaluation of Esophageal Sensation

Salman Nusrat, MD[a], Philip B. Miner Jr, MD[b],*

KEYWORDS

- Esophageal motility • Esophageal sensation
- High-resolution esophageal manometry • Multimodal esophageal assessment

KEY POINTS

- Dramatic progress has been made over the past decade in the sophistication and availability of equipment to test esophageal motility and sensation.
- High-resolution esophageal manometry and impedance have moved from the research clinic into clinical practice.
- Some of the testing is costly, time consuming, and requires extensive experience to perform the testing and properly interpret the results.
- The sensory studies are valuable in the interpretation of clinical problems, and provide important research information.
- Clinicians should evaluate the research studies to advance their understanding of the pathophysiology of the esophagus.

INTRODUCTION

Hippocrates noted in patients with "nausea, heartburn and salivation, there will be vomiting," setting the stage for exploring the relationship of esophageal sensory phenomena with pathophysiology of esophageal disease.[1] These 8 words capture the concepts of esophageal pain as an important clinical symptom, the bidirectional relationship of peripheral sensation and central nervous system response with nausea and vomiting, the complex gastrointestinal neurologic relationship of the esophagus and the stomach also causing vomiting, the relationship of esophageal sensation and sialorrhea, and the spectrum of gastroesophageal reflux from heartburn to vomiting. Rigorous clinical tests of esophageal sensation began nearly 6 decades ago with balloon distension, an exploration of referred pain locations associated with well-localized balloon placement throughout the gastrointestinal tract.[2] The

a Section of Digestive Disease and Nutrition, Department of Medicine, University of Oklahoma Health Sciences Center, Oklahoma City, OK 73104, USA; b Division of Gastroenterology, Department of Medicine, Oklahoma Foundation for Digestive Research, Oklahoma University School of Medicine, 525 Northwest 9th Street, Suite 325, Oklahoma City, OK 73102, USA
* Corresponding author.
E-mail address: philip-miner@ofdr.com

Gastrointest Endoscopy Clin N Am 24 (2014) 619–632
http://dx.doi.org/10.1016/j.giec.2014.06.005
1052-5157/14/$ – see front matter © 2014 Elsevier Inc. All rights reserved.

esophageal findings were simple. The location of discomfort with balloon distension is always at or proximal to the anatomic location of the balloon distension. This simple experiment provided the explanation for the clinical observation that an obstructive bolus at the gastroesophageal junction may present as discomfort from near the suprasternal notch to the gastroesophageal junction. Awareness of the importance of gastric acid as a cause of esophageal discomfort opened new vistas in drug development. To evaluate the role of acid in inducing esophageal symptoms, hydrochloric acid was infused into the esophagus to test the sensitivity of the esophagus to acid (Bernstein test). Measurement of endogenous esophageal acid exposure associated with gastroesophageal reflux with continuous esophageal pH measurements began with a bedside pH monitoring platform and evolved into ambulatory 24-hour pH recordings documenting gastric and esophageal pH with concurrent symptom recording. The amazing resolution of symptoms and esophageal erosions associated with control of gastric acid secretion and esophageal acid exposure gave birth to the hypothesis that all heartburn could be explained by acid secretion, with nonerosive esophageal reflux disease simply exposure to acid at a lower level than the acid exposure associated with erosive esophagitis. This hypothesis began to flounder with the recognition that excellent acid secretory control did not improve symptoms in many patients with nonerosive gastroesophageal reflux disease. As the drugs used to control acid secretion have achieved generic status, a new era in understanding esophageal pathophysiology has emerged with the proposal of alternative hypotheses to explain esophageal symptoms. Many of the hypotheses are based on the physiology and pathophysiology of sensation. Contemporary research in esophageal physiology and pathophysiology carries more interest, innovation, and importance than ever before. Evaluation of esophageal sensation plays an essential role in these research efforts.

NEUROPHYSIOLOGY OF THE ESOPHAGUS

Normal and aberrant sensory function are critical neurophysiologic components of esophageal function and pathophysiology. A simple inventory of common symptoms including the discomfort from a spoonful of peanut butter that doesn't seem to move, chest pain with a frozen drink, sialorrhea after the first sip of hot tea, the cough associated with vomiting, and symptoms of regurgitation or heartburn attests to the complexity of esophageal neurophysiology.

The required anatomic and physiologic transition from skeletal muscles controlled by somatic nerves to the smooth muscles innervated by the autonomic nervous system further emphasizes the complexity of neurophysiologic control of the esophagus.

In addition, sensory discrimination is perplexing, as intraesophageal balloon inflation occurs as either chest pain or heartburn irrespective of balloon volume or location. The quality of symptom perception may be independent of stimulus.[3]

Esophageal sensory testing focuses on understanding the differences in sensory perception in the proximal and distal esophagus, the role of the enteric nervous system in sensory perception, the role of the physiologic stress-response system in stimulus perception, the importance of the neuroimmune axis with the associated subset of inflammatory and immunologically induced pain pathways, and the relative importance of pain amplification pathways and central processing of abnormal esophageal sensation.

Efforts to understand the important details of these concepts have generated the development of the techniques described in this section on sensory testing of the esophagus. A recent article summarizes the state of the art of neurophysiologic research in esophageal physiology.[4]

GASTROINTESTINAL SENSITIVITY AND GASTROESOPHAGEAL REFLUX DISEASE

Prompt improvement of heartburn with antacid treatment suggests a direct relationship between acid in the esophagus and esophageal discomfort. Early clinical studies supported the importance of esophageal acid exposure and esophageal pain. In 1958, Bernstein and Baker[5] perfused 0.1 N HCl into the esophagus to identify patients with acid-induced esophagitis. The provocation of heartburn with the perfusion of the esophagus with acid became the first easily available test of esophageal sensitivity. The ability to monitor esophageal pH for 24 hours while signaling a symptomatic event onto the electronic pH record was an important advancement in the testing of esophageal sensitivity. Although the percent time of esophageal acid exposure to gastric fluid with a pH lower than 4.0 helps identify patients with symptomatic heartburn amenable to inhibition of gastric acid, the lack of association between symptoms and discrete acid reflux events failed to provide a convincing relationship between symptoms to a specific reflux event.[6] One explanation for the failure to correlate reflux events with symptoms is the observation that the more proximal the reflux event travels, the more likely a sensory stimulus will occur.

As an important corollary to the discordant pH recording and symptomatic events, the dissociation of the controlled perfusion of acid into the esophagus and the identification of abnormal esophageal acid exposure in patients with noncardiac chest pain (NCCP) challenges the paradigm that sensory perception of esophageal acid exposure is an easily interpretable event. Jung and colleagues[7] failed to find an association between symptoms induced by spontaneous reflux during prolonged esophageal pH monitoring and symptoms as a result of esophageal acid perfusion in patients with symptomatic heartburn, suggesting that the pathways of sensitivity in spontaneous esophageal acid exposure and provocative testing arise from different stimulatory pathways.

Prolonged monitoring of reflux events with impedance monitoring provides additional insight into the movement of fluid in the esophagus. The simultaneous measurement of esophageal pH and impedance support a role for pH and volume clearance time in symptomatic reflux events. Perception of volume plays an important role in esophageal sensation in normal subjects and in disease. Unfortunately, although impedance studies can determine the proximal extent of a reflux event, the technology is not yet able to provide information about the volume of refluxant into the esophagus, making it necessary to use the proximal location of refluxant as a surrogate marker for volume.

Although there is a clear clinical relationship between esophageal acid exposure and symptoms of heartburn, the temporal association of symptoms with a reflux event is perplexing. Addressing the difficulty of the poor symptom index with documented acid reflux has led to the numerous tests of esophageal sensitivity available today, in addition to sound paradigms for multiple sensory pathways, changes in permeability of the esophageal mucosa, and models of visceral hypersensitivity associated with molecular and inflammatory pathways. The discussion of esophageal sensitivity always begins with gastroesophageal reflux disease (GERD).

Independent of the evaluation of reflux events, extensive research focusing on molecular aspects of pain-induction pathways (the acid receptor TRPV1 and adenosine triphosphate, and the purine and pyrimidine receptor subfamilies P1, P2X, and P2Y) provides new information about esophageal sensitivity, and should lead to the development of new drugs for the management of esophageal pain.[8]

ESOPHAGEAL SENSITIVITY TESTING
Esophageal Manometry and 24-Hour Esophageal pH/Impedance

The important details of esophageal manometry and 24-hour pH/impedance are presented elsewhere in this issue. The assessment of esophageal sensitivity depends on these tests to provide important information about esophageal motor function and the exposure of the esophageal lumen to gastric contents.

Provocative Esophageal Perfusion Testing

The Bernstein esophageal acid perfusion test has a long history, recently fraught with controversy. The authors use a modified Bernstein test with a 5-minute saline infusion followed by 10 minutes of acid infusion. The initial sensation, discomfort, and pain thresholds are identified separately, and descriptors of the sensation are recorded in the patient's words. For a test to be positive, "typical symptoms" (symptoms for which the patient is being evaluated) need to be voiced, and the intensity of discomfort is recorded. The initial placebo control infusion period may be positive for typical symptoms, which may be due to sensitivity of the slightly acidic pH of unbuffered saline or sensitivity to fluid at room temperature. When the acid is perfused, the 3 thresholds of sensation are identified and the accompanying symptoms recorded. The authors use acid perfusion as an index of chemical sensitivity. As expected, most of the reported symptoms revolve around a description related to acid heartburn; however, approximately 16% of subjects report the symptom associated with acid infusion as "pressure," the symptom associated with balloon distension with testing or esophageal motor dysfunction by clinical history. Although the clinical value of provocative clinical testing may be an issue in the clinical assessment of GERD, chemical testing is a necessary part of the sensory assessment of esophageal function.

Of all of the esophageal perfusion provocative tests the authors have explored, the comparison of chenodeoxycholic acid and ursodeoxycholic acid has been the most interesting.[9] Using a complex infusion protocol, asymptomatic controls and patients with functional heartburn were given provocative esophageal sensory testing with 0.1 N HCl, 2 mM solutions of both ultrapure chenodeoxycholic and ursodeoxycholic acid (provided by Axcan Pharmaceuticals, Montreal, QC, Canada). If there was no reported pain after 15 minutes of esophageal perfusion of the bile acid (10 mL/min), the concentration of bile acid was increased to 5 mM for a maximum of 15 more minutes. Relative sensitivity to pain was greater with 0.1 N hydrochloric acid than with chenodeoxycholic acid, which was greater than with ursodeoxycholic acid. The difficulty in obtaining ultrapure bile acids prohibits utilization of esophageal perfusion of bile acids as a routine clinical test. This provocative sensory testing contributes the following to the understanding of esophageal sensation: (1) perfusion of the esophagus with the most prevalent bile acid (chenodeoxycholic acid) in lower concentration (2 mM) than is often found in the stomach of patients with enterogastric reflux (4 mM) causes heartburn symptoms; (2) different bile acids have different thresholds for provoking pain, with chenodeoxycholic acid more potent than ursodeoxycholic acid; and (3) using ursodeoxycholic acid to decrease chenodeoxycholic acid concentration in the bile acid pool may provide a therapeutic pathway for patients with bile reflux esophageal symptoms. The use of esophageal perfusion with specific chemical substances to test chemically activated sensory pathways should be considered in investigative studies exploring the pathophysiology of pain, and there may be limited value for specific clinical problems.

As a variant of provocative esophageal perfusion testing, the authors administered capsules containing capsaicin to patients with heartburn to test esophageal sensitivity to capsaicin before a standard reflux-inducing meal.[10] Directed delivery of capsaicin to the stomach assured that any symptoms induced by capsaicin would be related to gastroesophageal reflux and not oropharyngeal or esophageal symptoms arising from contact with capsaicin during swallowing. No change in the intensity of the symptoms occurred, but there was a dramatic shift in the time to heartburn, suggesting a sensitizing effect of the capsaicin. This clinical study was conducted around the time that transient receptor vanilloid potential (TRVP1) was recognized as a receptor for capsaicin, providing clinical relevance for the observation in animal studies that TRPV1 induced sensitization of the esophagus to gastroesophageal reflux of acid.[11]

The provocative chemical sensory testing discussed thus far has focused on sensory stimulatory pathways to classes of compounds. Specific food stimulation may also be used for exploring changes in esophageal physiology in individual patients. The authors evaluated a patient with pheasant-induced dysphagia who presented with severe chest pain and dysphagia every autumn for several years.[12] Esophageal biopsies demonstrated high numbers of eosinophils. The history suggested that the symptoms were related to a pheasant rice casserole. Esophageal motility and barium swallow studies were performed with the casserole prepared with and without the pheasant, documenting the occurrence of clinical symptoms and motility changes related to the pheasant component of the casserole. At the time of this provocative testing, eosinophilic esophagitis had not emerged as an important esophageal disease. As eosinophilic esophagitis has become better understood, there is no need for specific food testing in the presence of increased esophageal eosinophils. This innovative provocative test demonstrates the feasibility of specific testing for dietary sensory or immune-associated symptoms.

Noncardiac Chest Pain Provocative Testing

NCCP refers to symptomatic chest pain, which has been evaluated and for which a cardiac cause has been excluded. The second tier of evaluation explores esophageal pain as the cause of the chest pain. In a recent large multicenter study, 70% of the patients with NCCP had normal esophageal manometry.[13] Richter and colleagues[14] compared the acid perfusion test with 24-hour esophageal pH monitoring, and found pH monitoring to be a superior diagnostic test for identification of an acid-sensitive esophagus in NCCP patients.

Some patients with chest pain of esophageal origin may be identified only by provocative testing during esophageal manometry. Edrophonium is an anticholinesterase with a short half-life and onset of action within 60 seconds. London and colleagues[15] showed that the administration of ergonovine or edrophonium provoked typical chest pain in association with high amplitude, long duration, and repetitive esophageal contractions in all patients. However, none of the controls in their study reported chest pain in response to ergonovine or edrophonium. The test can be performed by injecting either 80 mg/kg or 10 mg/kg followed by 5 to 10 swallows of 5 to 10 mL of water over 5 to 10 minutes. The routine use of provocative testing for chest pain in clinical practice is limited by the fact that these drugs can induce coronary spasms, and are associated with other side effects related to excessive cholinergic stimulation such as increased salivation and abdominal cramps.

Techniques such as functional magnetic resonance imaging (fMRI), positron emission tomography (PET), magnetoencephalography, and electroencephalography have led to the identification of a network of brain areas that processes visceral sensation. These studies have improved understanding of the pathophysiology of NCCP, and are discussed in more detail later.

Provocative Barostat Balloon Testing

Balloon distension testing of sensation in the gastrointestinal tract has been used for decades to investigate the physiology and pathophysiology of the gastrointestinal tract. Latex balloons and hand-held syringes were used until the advent of the electronic barostat. Latex balloons were chosen because of the low profile when deflated, the low cost (condoms), and the tolerance of latex to very large volumes of distension. When intraballoon pressure became an important experimental end point of esophageal balloon distension, the hysteresis and nonlinear elasticity of the latex became a disadvantage as the intrinsic pressure of the inflated latex balloon at each distension volume needed to be subtracted from the measured pressure, and pressure profiles of the balloon could change with each inflation, making accurate pressure readings impossible. Because the pressure curves of pressure against volume (compliance) are not linear, calculations and interpretations of data acquired with latex balloon distension were difficult. This difficulty led to the inflation of an infinitely compliant balloon with no intrinsic wall pressure using an electronically controlled barostat. The barostat controls balloon pressure and simultaneously measures balloon volume. Although the barostat has become the instrument of choice for luminal pressure and distension studies, diagnostic protocols and standard values are not widely available. Another serious issue unique to esophageal balloon placement concerns keeping the esophageal balloon in a designated location in the esophagus. The ellipsoid latex balloon is pulled toward the stomach with strong longitudinal force, often entering into the stomach, which complicates interpretation of the data. Approximately 10 years ago the authors developed a cylindrical, infinitely compliant balloon with a slippery synthetic surface (**Fig. 1**) that allows the balloon to stay in place in the esophagus with little longitudinal force. The current research trend is to use intraballoon pressure (mm Hg), rather than balloon volume (milliliters of air), as the quantitative measure to assess sensitivity. Barlow and colleagues[16] investigated esophageal distension with manometry and impedance planimetry to demonstrate that stretch and not tension activated the sense of distension in normal subjects. In the assessment of patients with visceral hypersensitivity, the authors can demonstrate sensitivity to both pressure and volume, often independently, suggesting multiple sensory distortion pathways for abnormalities of visceral sensation. Because the authors have postulated that stretch (volume in milliliters) and pressure (mm Hg) receptors may have variable sensitivity, their data are reported with both volume and pressure. Three symptom end points are assessed: first sensation, discomfort, and pain. In the authors' clinical practice and research studies, the balloon is placed above the lower esophageal sphincter and below the upper esophageal sphincter for 2 separate inflation studies to assess the differences in proximal and distal sensory function.

To visualize the data obtained from esophageal barostat studies, the last control cohort is presented in **Table 1**.

Difficulties often arise in discussing barostat data between studies because of the absence of standard sensory assessment protocols, differences in balloon shapes,

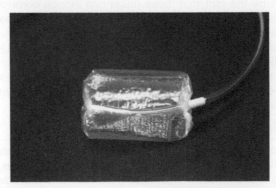

Fig. 1. The cylindrical, infinitely compliant balloon developed by the authors.

Table 1 Data from esophageal barostat studies				
	UES Pressure	UES Volume	LES Pressure	LES Volume
First sensation				
Males	12.7 ± 7.1	8.1 ± 5.5	16.5 ± 8.8	12.8 ± 7.6
Females	5.7 ± 5	4.0 ± 2.1	9.1 ± 6.2	6 ± 3.3
Discomfort				
Males	25.5 ± 14.5	18.1 ± 12.6	32.2 ± 15.5	18.1 ± 12.5
Females	14.0 ± 6.4	9.4 ± 2.7	16.4 ± 5.8	12.9 ± 4.14
Pain				
Males	41.2 ± 13.7	38.8 ± 17.7	47.8 ± 13.7	48.4 ± 17.4
Females	24.5 ± 13.1	20.0 ± 11.1	30.0 ± 11.7	24.4 ± 11.1

Pressure is recorded as mm Hg and volume is in mL of air in the balloon.

construction of balloons with different materials, and quantitative differences in balloon hysteresis and nonlinear elasticity. The data in **Table 1** are derived from normal subjects used to establish the values in the authors' laboratory, and specific means and standard deviations cannot be used for other clinical or research laboratories. Important concepts derived from such normal studies include the relationship of volume and pressure tolerance, the differences in sensation between the proximal and distal esophagus, and gender differences. The gender differences are particularly dramatic, with every gender comparison having significance with P values of less than .006, although the gender difference has not been confirmed by others.[17] If gender differences are demonstrated by additional studies, the implications for functional gastrointestinal disease and sensory testing, clinically and for drug development, are profound, and may explain the gender differences observed in the conduct of clinical trials in functional diseases.

Impedance Planimetry

Impedance planimetry provides an alternative esophageal distension technique using 0.018% saline and a pressure-leveling system. By moving the leveling chamber in the vertical plane, the amount of water in the esophageal balloon changes as the balloon pressure changes. The density of the 0.018% saline is so close to the density of water that recording the pressure results as centimeters of water is satisfactory. The importance of the saline is to provide an ionic environment capable of conducting the electric current, which is necessary to assess impedance values used to calculate cross-sectional area. This technique not only provides an assessment of the cross-sectional area of the lumen in a selected plane but also permits quantification of the resistance offered by the viscoelastic properties of the wall and the phasic contractions of the muscle, and provides an assessment of the visceral sensory responses that occur during balloon distension.[18–20] Measurement of balloon volume at the predetermined sensory end points is possible by direct measurement of the volume of saline in the balloon and by mathematical calculation using the cross-sectional area. One of the values of this technique is the ability to measure changes in luminal cross-sectional area associated with esophageal accommodation and peristaltic contraction along the length of the balloon. Volume of the balloon is generally not reported. One of the early clinical studies using this technique confirmed its usefulness by demonstrating that patients with chest pain and normal cardiac and esophageal evaluations had reproduction of their symptoms with impedance planimetry associated with a lower sensory threshold for pain and reduced esophageal compliance.[21] The same research group compared impedance planimetry with the barostat, demonstrating similar data regarding sensory perception, esophageal wall distensibility, and biomechanical properties. The purported advantage of dynamic balloon distension (the distension technique used for impedance planimetry) was better tolerance of the procedure.[22] The sensory standards from the authors' normal subjects closely match the pressure values and sensory end points in these studies. The development of high-resolution impedance planimetry probes provides an opportunity to obtain more detailed evaluation of esophageal distensibility, thus helping to correlate the biomechanical properties of the esophagus with sensory changes.[23]

Multimodal Esophageal Assessment

Recently a multimodal esophageal assessment catheter has been developed, which uses a single catheter to assess, singly or simultaneously, mechanical, electrical, chemical, heat, and cold stimulation of the esophagus.[24] The development of this catheter arose from the neurophysiologic construct that multiple sensory inputs are simultaneously processed to generate esophageal sensation. Sensory evaluation of patients with erosive esophagitis, nonerosive gastroesophageal reflux disease, functional chest pain, and Barrett esophagus confirmed the reliability of the data acquired from the probe.[24–29] Some of the findings of these and other studies are summarized in **Table 2**.[30] At present, there is little experience with either of these interesting techniques apart from that of the developmental teams.

Esophageal Evoked Potentials

The techniques described thus far rely predominantly on subjective reporting of pain ratings, and therefore are susceptible to response bias and are incapable of objectively dissociating between the potential candidate mechanisms of visceral hypersensitivity.

Cortical neural activity can be recorded in real time using magnetoencephalography and electroencephalography. It is now well established that when magnetoencephalography and electroencephalography are recorded in response to repetitive esophageal stimulation, highly reproducible esophageal evoked potentials (EEPs) can be recorded. EEPs represent the sequence of voltage changes within the brain that occurs after an esophageal stimulus, and is a robust method that provides objective, stimulus-specific neural measures of esophageal afferent pathway sensitivity. EEPs can be used to determine the neurophysiologic characteristics of esophageal afferent pathways, detect changes in the sensitivity of these afferents after experimental acidification, and identify the cortical neural correlates of each EEP component.[31]

Table 2
Sensation alterations in patients with esophageal disorders as measured by multimodal esophageal assessment

	Acid	Distension	Heat	Central Sensitization
ERD	Increased	Decreased	Increased	Increased
NERD	Increased	Decreased	Increased	Increased
Barrett esophagus	Decreased	Decreased	Decreased	Unchanged
NCCP	Increased	Increased	N/A	Increased
EoE	Increased	Unchanged	Unchanged	Unchanged

Abbreviations: EoE, eosinophilic esophagitis; ERD, esophageal reflux disease; N/A, not applicable; NCCP, noncardiac chest pain; NERD, nonerosive reflux disease.

Electrical stimulation and balloon distension have been use to assess cerebral evoked potential, but at present it is unclear whether one is superior to the other. Balloon distension triggers a triphasic evoked potential comprising 2 negative peaks (N1 and N2) and 1 positive peak (P1).[32] Each component of the EEP relates to a specific step in the processing of esophageal sensory information, that is, all of the processing from stimulus activation in the esophagus to the cerebral cortex. Latency is defined as the time from the stimulus to the peak. NCCP patients with reduced pain thresholds can present with reduced or normal latency suggestive of either heightened peripheral pathway sensitivity or increased cerebral processing, respectively.[31] Cerebral evoked potentials provided the opportunity to separate out exogenous cortical responses (stimulus-dependent activity) from endogenous responses. Activity that occurs after more than 300 milliseconds represents endogenous cortical activity, whereas the activity that occurs up to approximately 300 milliseconds after stimulation represents the exogenous component of esophageal-cortical sensory processing.[33,34]

Brain Imaging

The neuroanatomic localization of the stimulated area of the brain during esophageal stimulation may be determined using fMRI and PET.[35] PET depends on detecting positron-emitting radionuclides that are injected intravenously while the subject's head is positioned in a specialized detection system. Regional cerebral blood flow has been shown to correlate with neuronal activity[36] and, based on this principle, PET uses radiolabeled compounds to create tomographic images that measure blood flow to the brain. The most commonly used radiolabeled compound in gastrointestinal research is ^{15}O, which is prepared as $H_2^{15}O$-labeled water, but currently there are hundreds of radiolabeled compounds used in PET, each with their own characteristics and used for imaging particular biochemical or physiologic processes.[37,38]

One of the first studies to describe the pain neuromatrix activated by gastrointestinal stimulation used PET to compare cortical activation patterns with nonpainful and painful esophageal stimuli,[39] using a relatively simple block-design paradigm whereby subtraction analysis was used to compare 3 conditions: no sensation, nonpainful sensation, and pain. The resultant images demonstrated that nonpainful esophageal stimulation elicited bilateral activation of the primary/secondary somatosensory cortex and insula. Painful esophageal stimulation, as one would expect, not only led to increased activity within these regions but also activated the anterior cingulate cortex.

fMRI produces images of active brain regions by detecting indirect effects of neural activity on local blood flow, volume, and oxygen saturation, giving detailed information regarding the functional neuroanatomy of the brain.[38] The most commonly used fMRI technique relies on the detection of naturally occurring differences in the magnetic properties of blood constituents, namely deoxygenated hemoglobin, which because of its paramagnetic properties within the blood can identify changes in its regional distribution during conditions that change neuronal activation.[38] fMRI was used by Kern and colleagues[40] to evaluate the activation of cerebral cortex in response to esophageal acid exposure (0.1 N HCl) in healthy controls. These investigators noted that cerebral cortical activity was concentrated in the posterior cingulate, parietal, and anteromesial frontal lobes. The superior frontal lobe regions activated during their study corresponded to Brodmann area 32, the insula, the operculum, and the anterior cingulate. The same group later reported that cortical activity occurs with greater intensity and more rapidly in GERD patients than the activity in response to subliminal acid exposure in healthy controls.[41]

As noted earlier, similar patterns of cortical activation can be observed in the presence or absence of peripheral stimuli,[42] and PET and fMRI currently do not have sufficient temporal resolution to separate exogenous and endogenous cortical activity, therefore making interpretation of these data difficult. In addition, high cost and prolonged assessment time limit the use of fMRI and PET to research activities designed to better understand the details of central processing of esophageal sensory information.

Immunologically Mediated Sensory Pathways

The concept of immune-mediated gastrointestinal pain emerged in the early phase of understanding of the neuroimmune axis. The conceptual model arose in an attempt to explain functional gastrointestinal pain that began with a discrete event, enteric infection. Now identified as postinfectious irritable bowel syndrome (IBS), the initial observation was made in 1962 by Chaudhary and Truelove[43] with the onset of IBS in British vacationers to Spain. In the 1980s, interest in gastrointestinal mast cells eventually led to numerous basic science and clinical studies tying the central nervous system activation of immunologic response with a bidirectional component in which gastrointestinal immune activation signaled the central nervous system. In a small number of patients known to have high numbers of mast cells in their gastrointestinal tract, dramatic sensitivity to rectal balloon distension was so close to data in IBS patients that the linkage of the immune system, specifically mast cells, to IBS became a working hypothesis for IBS visceral sensitivity. Esophageal symptoms of discomfort and pain are linked to inflammation. In addition, inflammation sensitizes afferent nerve terminals through associated changes in esophageal permeability. Permeability changes are proposed to allow access of acid to the submucosa, inducing chemical sensitization. Transient receptor potential vanilloid (TRPV1) influences esophageal sensation (vide supra). TRPV1 is gated by heat and acid, which leads to activation of platelet-activating factor (PAF).[44] PAF is a chemoattractant and activator of immune cells. The upregulation of proteinase-activated receptor 2 and the expression of interleukin-8 in esophageal biopsies from patients with nonerosive reflux disease support the proposed immunologic pathway as being one of the mechanisms of esophageal hypersensitivity.[45]

The best-recognized immune-related esophageal disease associated with esophageal visceral hypersensitivity is eosinophilic esophagitis. Although dysphagia and food impaction occur more often than chest pain or heartburn, chest pain and discomfort are common in patients with eosinophilic esophagitis. In a recent publication exploring the incidence of esophageal eosinophil infiltration in patients with noncardiac chest pain, Achem and colleagues[46] found 14% of their NCCP cohort had elevated eosinophil counts in the esophageal mucosa. This observation suggests that chest pain may be one of the primary symptoms manifested by patients with eosinophilic esophagitis. Several eosinophilic causes of esophageal pain sensations are possible in these patients, including motor changes associated with a poorly compliant esophagus, the tissue changes found in the esophagus secondary to the inflammatory action of eosinophils, and immune-mediated pain. Immune-activated pain is complex and is poorly responsive to narcotic pain medication protocols. Primary sensory activation through changes in immune function form one of the major components of the neuroimmune axis, with bidirectional communication of central nervous system signals activating mast cell and eosinophil function, as well as with primary activation of the immune system. The immune linkage of eosinophils with esophageal symptoms was demonstrated in the pheasant-induced dysphagia before recognition and acceptance of this disorder, now recognized as eosinophilic esophagitis.[12] As advances in understanding the role of immune stimulation in visceral sensitivity advance, assessment of gastrointestinal immune disorders will become a routine part of the assessment of esophageal visceral hyperalgesia.

Implications for Esophageal Sensory Testing in Understanding the Pathophysiology of Esophageal Disease and in Drug Development

In the course of the discussion regarding testing esophageal sensation, the articles mentioned have alluded to many new physiologic and pathophysiologic aspects of the esophagus. Two specific examples of the exploration of esophageal sensation may inspire sensory evaluation studies in the research setting and clinical practice. Tegaserod is a serotonin receptor 4 (5-HT$_4$) partial agonist that was briefly approved for the treatment of IBS. The 5-HT receptors play an active role in gastrointestinal sensitization, and the success of tegaserod in IBS suggested a sensory improvement in colonic symptoms. The ubiquitous importance of serotonin in the gastrointestinal tract led to the hypothesis that tegaserod may be useful in modifying esophageal sensitization. A protocol was designed to test alteration of mechanical (barostat) and chemical (Bernstein test) sensitivity associated with the administration of tegaserod in patients with functional heartburn. Tegaserod significantly improved clinical symptoms of heartburn/acid reflux, regurgitation, and distress from regurgitation. The barostat study end points of balloon pressure to pain and wall tension improved significantly, and the pain with acid perfusion was not changed. The effect on the mechanical sensitivity threshold without altering the chemical sensitivity threshold suggests 2 distinct sensory pathways with different pharmacologic response patterns.[47] The opposite pattern of sensory improvement was seen with esophageal sensitivity studies using the H2-receptor antagonist (H2RA) ranitidine. With the simultaneous release of cimetidine and sucralfate for ulcer disease in 1976, cimetidine outperformed sucralfate in the marketplace despite nearly equivalent ulcer-healing efficacy. One of the remarkable clinical findings was the decrease in pain following the initiation of cimetidine treatment before resolution of the ulcer, which occurred before pain improvement with sucralfate. The hypothesis that H2RAs influenced gastrointestinal sensation was promulgated in the early 1980s, with funding of the research granted in the early 2000s. In a functional heartburn population, barostat and Bernstein testing were performed with ranitidine 150 mg as a single dose and after 7 days of twice-daily dosing. The response to exogenous acid perfusion was significantly different after a single dose, with no tachyphylaxis after 7 days. There was no effect on mechanical sensitivity.[48] The ability of esophageal sensory testing to demonstrate different sensory responses that may be modified separately opens new vistas in the understanding of normal esophageal physiology and the pathophysiology of esophageal disease. Sophisticated sensory testing has become an important area of gastrointestinal research.

Current Clinical Assessment Recommendations

Dramatic progress has been made over the past decade in the sophistication and availability of equipment to test esophageal motility and sensation. High-resolution esophageal manometry and impedance have moved from the research clinic onto the on-ramp of clinical practice. This technological advance has changed the conceptual model of normal esophageal motility and the understanding of esophageal pathophysiology in ways that could never have been predicted. The focus on sensory testing is limited to research laboratories at present. Some of the testing is costly and time consuming, and requires extensive experience to perform the testing and properly interpret the results. Uniform testing procedures and equipment need to be established before the technology can become available to the clinician, either through referral to a tertiary care center or by providing local and easily utilized diagnostic platforms for practice/hospital use. For the last decade the authors have performed Bernstein and barostat testing as part of their esophageal manometry studies in nearly all patients. The sensory studies are valuable in the interpretation of clinical problems, and provide important research information. Sensory testing at this level is a luxury for patients and will not be easily available in the foreseeable future. Clinicians should evaluate the research studies to advance their understanding of the pathophysiology of the esophagus. Moreover, they should demand that publications clearly state the patient population and publish clinical characteristics of the population that may provide clinical recognition of the disorder being discussed, and articulate the research findings in a practical and clinically applicable style. The academic camp of esophagologists faces many challenges, but this field has never been more intellectually stimulating or clinically rewarding.

REFERENCES

1. Potter P, Jones WH. Coan prenotions-Anatomical and Minor Clinical Writing. In: Potter P, editor. Hippocrates, vol. IX. Cambridge, MA: Harvard University Press; 2010. p. 135.
2. Lipkin M, Sleisenger MH. Studies of visceral pain: measurements of stimulus intensity and duration associated with the onset of pain in esophagus, ileum and colon. J Clin Invest 1958;37(1):28.
3. Fass R, Naliboff B, Higa L, et al. Differential effect of long-term esophageal acid exposure on mechanosensitivity and chemosensitivity in humans. Gastroenterology 1998;115(6):1363–73.
4. Woodland P, Sifrim D, Krarup AL, et al. The neurophysiology of the esophagus. Ann N Y Acad Sci 2013;1300(1):53–70.
5. Bernstein L, Baker LA. A clinical test for esophagitis. Gastroenterology 1958; 34(5):760–81.
6. Cicala M, Emerenziani S, Caviglia R, et al. Intra-oesophageal distribution and perception of acid reflux in patients with non-erosive gastro-oesophageal reflux disease. Aliment Pharmacol Therapeut 2003;18(6):605–13.
7. Jung B, Steinbach J, Beaumont C, et al. Lack of association between esophageal acid sensitivity detected by prolonged pH monitoring and Bernstein testing. Am J Gastroenterol 2004;99(3):410–5.
8. Altomare A, Guarino L, Pier M, et al. Gastrointestinal sensitivity and gastroesophageal reflux disease. Ann N Y Acad Sci 2013;1300(1):80–95.
9. Siddiqui A, Rodriguez-Stanley S, Zubaidi S, et al. Esophageal visceral sensitivity to bile salts in patients with functional heartburn and in healthy control subjects. Dig Dis Sci 2005;50(1):81–5.
10. Rodriguez-Stanley S, Collings K, Robinson M, et al. The effects of capsaicin on reflux, gastric emptying and dyspepsia. Aliment Pharmacol Ther 2000;14: 129–34.
11. Szallasi A, Blumberg PM. Vanilloid (capsaicin) receptors and mechanisms. Pharmacol Rev 1999;51(2):159–212.
12. Rodriguez-Stanley S, Robinson M, Biscopink RJ, et al. Case report: pheasant-induced dysphagia. Dig Dis Sci 2000;45(9):1743–6.
13. Dekel R, Pearson T, Wendel C, et al. Assessment of oesophageal motor function in patients with dysphagia or chest pain—the Clinical outcomes research initiative experience. Aliment Pharmacol Therapeut 2003;18(11-12):1083–9.

14. Richter JE, Hewson EG, Sinclair JW, et al. Acid perfusion test and 24-hour esophageal pH monitoring with symptom index. Dig Dis Sci 1991;36(5):565–71.
15. London R, Ouyang A, Snape W, et al. Provocation of esophageal pain by ergonovine or edrophonium. Gastroenterology 1981;81(1):10–4.
16. Barlow JD, Gregersen H, Thompson DG. Identification of the biomechanical factors associated with the perception of distension in the human esophagus. Am J Physiol Gastrointest Liver Physiol 2002;282(4):G683–9.
17. Rao SS, Mudipalli RS, Mujica VR, et al. Effects of gender and age on esophageal biomechanical properties and sensation. Am J Gastroenterol 2003;98(8): 1688–95.
18. Gregersen H, Andersen M. Impedance measuring system for quantification of cross-sectional area in the gastrointestinal tract. Med Biol Eng Comput 1991; 29(1):108–10.
19. Gregersen H, Djurhuus J. Impedance planimetry: a new approach to biomechanical intestinal wall properties. Dig Dis 1991;9(6):332–40.
20. Rao SS, Hayek B, Summers RW. Impedance planimetry: an integrated approach for assessing sensory, active, and passive biomechanical properties of the human esophagus. Am J Gastroenterol 1995;90(3):431–8.
21. Rao SS, Gregersen H, Hayek B, et al. Unexplained chest pain: the hypersensitive, hyperreactive, and poorly compliant esophagus. Ann Intern Med 1996;124(11): 950–8.
22. Remes-Troche J, Attaluri A, Chahal P, et al. Barostat or dynamic balloon distention test: which technique is best suited for esophageal sensory testing? Dis Esophagus 2012;25(7):584–9.
23. Nicodème F, Hirano I, Chen J, et al. Esophageal distensibility as a measure of disease severity in patients with eosinophilic esophagitis. Clin Gastroenterol Hepatol 2013;11(9):1101–7.e1.
24. Drewes AM, Schipper KP, Dimcevski G, et al. Multimodal assessment of pain in the esophagus: a new experimental model. Am J Physiol Gastrointest Liver Physiol 2002;283(1):G95–103.
25. Krarup AL, Olesen SS, Funch-Jensen P, et al. Proximal and distal esophageal sensitivity is decreased in patients with Barrett's esophagus. World J Gastroenterol 2011;17(4):514.
26. Krarup AL, Villadsen GE, Mejlgaard E, et al. Acid hypersensitivity in patients with eosinophilic oesophagitis. Scand J Gastroenterol 2010;45(3):273–81.
27. Krarup AL, Simrén M, Funch-Jensen P, et al. The esophageal multimodal pain model: normal values and degree of sensitization in healthy young male volunteers. Dig Dis Sci 2011;56(7):1967–75.
28. Reddy H, Staahl C, Arendt-Nielsen L, et al. Sensory and biomechanical properties of the esophagus in non-erosive reflux disease. Scand J Gastroenterol 2007;42(4):432–40.
29. Drewes AM, Reddy H, Pedersen J, et al. Multimodal pain stimulations in patients with grade B oesophagitis. Gut 2006;55(7):926–32.
30. McKemy DD, Neuhausser WM, Julius D. Identification of a cold receptor reveals a general role for TRP channels in thermosensation. Nature 2002;416(6876): 52–8.
31. Hobson AR, Furlong PL, Sarkar S, et al. Neurophysiologic assessment of esophageal sensory processing in noncardiac chest pain. Gastroenterology 2006; 130(1):80–8.
32. Smout A, DeVore M, Castell D. Cerebral potentials evoked by esophageal distension in human. Am J Physiol Gastrointest Liver Physiol 1990;259(6):G955–9.

33. Hobson AR, Furlong PL, Worthen SF, et al. Real-time imaging of human cortical activity evoked by painful esophageal stimulation. Gastroenterology 2005; 128(3):610–9.
34. Hollerbach S, Fitzpatrick D, Shine G, et al. Cognitive evoked potentials to anticipated oesophageal stimulus in humans: quantitative assessment of the cognitive aspects of visceral perception. Neurogastroenterol Motil 1999;11:37–46.
35. Belliveau J, Kennedy D, McKinstry R, et al. Functional mapping of the human visual cortex by magnetic resonance imaging. Science 1991;254(5032):716–9.
36. Heeger DJ, Ress D. What does fMRI tell us about neuronal activity? Nat Rev Neurosci 2002;3(2):142–51.
37. Papanicolaou AC. Fundamentals of functional brain imaging: a guide to the methods and their applications to psychology and behavioral neuroscience. Oxon, United Kingdom: Taylor & Francis; 1998.
38. Orrison WW. Functional brain imaging. Maryland Heights, MO: Mosby; 1995.
39. Aziz Q, Andersson J, Valind S, et al. Identification of human brain loci processing esophageal sensation using positron emission tomography. Gastroenterology 1997;113(1):50–9.
40. Kern MK, Birn RM, Jaradeh S, et al. Identification and characterization of cerebral cortical response to esophageal mucosal acid exposure and distention. Gastroenterology 1998;115(6):1353–62.
41. Kern M, Hofmann C, Hyde J, et al. Characterization of the cerebral cortical representation of heartburn in GERD patients. Am J Physiol Gastrointest Liver Physiol 2004;286(1):G174–81.
42. Derbyshire SW, Whalley MG, Stenger VA, et al. Cerebral activation during hypnotically induced and imagined pain. Neuroimage 2004;23(1):392–401.
43. Chaudhary NA, Truelove SC. The irritable colon syndrome a study of the clinical features, predisposing causes, and prognosis in 130 cases. QJM 1962;31(3): 307–22.
44. Ma J, Harnett KM, Behar J, et al. Signaling in TRPV1-induced platelet activating factor (PAF) in human esophageal epithelial cells. Am J Physiol Gastrointest Liver Physiol 2010;298(2):G233–40.
45. Kandulski A, Wex T, Mönkemüller K, et al. Proteinase-activated receptor-2 in the pathogenesis of gastroesophageal reflux disease. Am J Gastroenterol 2010; 105(9):1934–43.
46. Achem S, Almansa C, Krishna M, et al. Oesophageal eosinophilic infiltration in patients with noncardiac chest pain. Aliment Pharmacol Therapeut 2011; 33(11):1194–201.
47. Rodriguez–Stanley S, Zubaidi S, Proskin HM, et al. Effect of tegaserod on esophageal pain threshold, regurgitation, and symptom relief in patients with functional heartburn and mechanical sensitivity. Clin Gastroenterol Hepatol 2006;4(4): 442–50.
48. Rodriguez-Stanley S, Ciociola A, Zubaidi S, et al. A single dose of ranitidine 150 mg modulates oesophageal acid sensitivity in patients with functional heartburn. Aliment Pharmacol Therapeut 2004;20(9):975–82.

Utilization of Esophageal Function Testing for the Diagnosis of the Rumination Syndrome and Belching Disorders

Caroline M.G. Saleh, MS, Albert J. Bredenoord, MD*

KEYWORDS

• Rumination • Belching • Manometry • pH impedance • Diagnosis

KEY POINTS

- The underlying mechanism of rumination is characterized by an increase in intragastric pressure.
- Combined manometry and pH impedance are preferred to distinguish rumination and belching disorders from other esophageal pathologies.
- In supragastric belches air is expelled immediately after ingestion; it is often caused by contraction of the diaphragm, creating negative pressures in the thoracic cavity and esophagus.
- On impedance supragastric belches are observed as an increase in impedance, starting in the proximal channel, and progressing to a distal channel, followed by a return to baseline starting in the distal channel.
- Manometry is crucial for identification of rumination and other esophageal pathologies; however typical patterns of supragastric belches are better observed on impedance.

INTRODUCTION

Rumination is a phenomenon characterized by retrograde flow of gastric contents into the mouth, otherwise known as regurgitation.[1] Repetitive excessive occurrence of rumination is considered pathologic and is known as the rumination syndrome[2]; this is a behavioral disorder, first thought to be only present in children and mentally disabled but currently increasingly recognized in otherwise healthy adult patients as well.

Belching occurs occasionally in everyone and is often not related to a disease or a pathologic condition.[3] There are 2 types of belches: gastric belches and supragastric belches.[4] Gastric belches are physiologic events caused by retrograde flow of air into

Department of Gastroenterology and Hepatology, Academic Medical Center Amsterdam, Meibergdreef 9, Amsterdam 1105 AZ, The Netherlands
* Corresponding author.
E-mail address: a.j.bredenoord@amc.uva.nl

Gastrointest Endoscopy Clin N Am 24 (2014) 633–642
http://dx.doi.org/10.1016/j.giec.2014.06.002
1052-5157/14/$ – see front matter © 2014 Elsevier Inc. All rights reserved.

the esophagus and mouth; however supragastric belching is associated with belching disorders and is considered pathologic behavior.[3]

Clinical diagnosis of the rumination syndrome and belching disorders are based on the ROME III criteria, which strangely enough defines both diseases as functional gastroduodenal disorders.[5–7] Unfortunately, patients frequently suffer several years and often consult many different physicians before being diagnosed correctly[1,8]; this is partly because other diseases such as gastroesophageal reflux disease (GERD) show many similarities in symptomatology with the rumination syndrome and the excessive belching disorder.[5,9]

Fortunately, recent technological advances, such as high-resolution manometry (HRM) combined with impedance, have allowed us to facilitate the detection and diagnosis of the rumination syndrome and supragastric belching.

In this article, the authors aim to provide an overview of the current diagnostic tools to improve the recognition and diagnostic approach of the rumination syndrome and belching disorders. For better understanding, both disorders will be discussed separately.

THE RUMINATION SYNDROME
Pathophysiology

Rumination is the voluntary, albeit unconscious, contraction of the abdominal muscles forcing return of food into the mouth, followed by rechewing, swallowing, or spitting.[1,10] The underlying mechanism is characterized by an increase in intragastric pressure, as a result of gastric straining.[11,12] When the intragastric pressure overcomes the pressure of the lower esophageal sphincter (LES), gastric content can flow into the esophagus. As a result, relaxation of the upper esophageal sphincter (UES) occurs and gastric content can subsequently flow from the esophagus into the pharynx and mouth.[13] The reason for the relatively "lower" LES pressure is still unclear, but could be caused by a prolonged low LES pressure postprandially or a temporary lowering during transient LES relaxations (TLESRs), which are sensed by the subject.[14,15] A third hypothesis is a learned, voluntary relaxation of the diaphragmatic crura that allows the normal postprandial increase in intragastric pressure to overcome the resistance to retrograde flow provided by the LES.[15]

The reason for gastric straining in patients suffering from rumination is still unclear. A study conducted by Tucker and colleagues[1] has shown that rumination is often seen as a behavioral response to abdominal pain or other unpleasant digestive symptoms. However, other studies have also suggested that psychological factors, such as stressful life events, lead to rumination.[16]

Clinical Evaluation and Diagnostic Approach

Clinical evaluation of the rumination syndrome is based on the ROME III criteria and is defined as persistent or recurrent regurgitation of recently ingested food into the mouth with subsequent spitting or remastication and swallowing.[7] Patients suffering from rumination syndrome typically present themselves with regurgitation, starting during the meal or in the immediate postprandial period. Regurgitation of gastric contents may occur several times per minute and is often described as having the same taste and consistency as the consumed food.[8] Another commonly seen symptom is weight loss, which can occur in up to 83% of patients with the rumination syndrome.[17] Furthermore, the response to acid suppression is often limited or absent.[9]

Experienced clinicians can recognize patients with rumination syndrome by clinical observation alone. However, only a few physicians have significant experience because of the low prevalence of the syndrome. Thus, patients with rumination syndrome often present to physicians who have never seen a patient with the condition before. Furthermore, the clinical presentation of the rumination syndrome shows many similarities (such as regurgitation) with other conditions and is therefore often mistaken for diseases such as GERD, gastroparesis, and cyclic vomiting. Therefore, the diagnosis of the rumination syndrome is made on both clinical observation and physiologic measurements. Currently, it is preferred to use conventional manometry or HRM combined with pH impedance to distinguish rumination syndrome from belching/regurgitation disorders and GERD.[9,11]

With combined manometry (conventional/HRM) and pH impedance, 3 variations of the rumination syndrome can be identified: (1) rumination without any leading events (classic rumination), (2) rumination occurring exclusively after a reflux episode (reflux rumination or secondary rumination), and (3) rumination caused by air swallowing and subsequent gastric straining (supragastric rumination).[1,17,18] Each subtype has a specific pattern, which can be identified on manometry and impedance measurements. On manometry, classic rumination presents itself with a sharp increase in intragastric pressure, also known as the "R-wave", before gastric contents are returned into the mouth (**Figs. 1**A and **2**A). Reflux rumination is caused by a gastric strain that occurs following a TLESR with common cavity pressure, resulting in regurgitation of gastric contents. The manometry of a patient with reflux rumination will display a moment of LES pressure decrease (TLESR), which is not present in a patient with classic rumination (see **Figs. 1**B and **2**B). The third subtype, supragastric rumination, is caused by swallowed air and subsequent gastric straining, which is then used to drive esophageal contents into the mouth (ie, never passes into the stomach). In this case, the LES does not relax on manometry (see **Figs. 1**C and **2**C). As seen in the figures, each subtype of the rumination syndrome is characterized by an increase in intragastric pressure (gastric strain).[1] This increase in intragastric pressure is a very important characteristic to distinguish rumination from other disorders such as GERD.[17] A study conducted by Kessing and colleagues[17] showed that 70% of patients with rumination exhibited gastric pressure peaks of greater than 30 mm Hg preceding the retrograde gastroesophageal flow, whereas 0% of patients with GERD presented peaks of greater than 30 mm Hg, demonstrating that with the 30 mm Hg cutoff a specificity of 100% was obtained.

The study conducted by Kessing and colleagues[17] also investigated the value of 24-hour pH impedance without manometry, in distinguishing rumination from other disorders. The result was that on average in rumination patients a higher percentage of reflux episodes reached the proximal esophagus; thus this finding alone was not sufficient to differentiate rumination from GERD. However, as **Fig. 1** demonstrates, impedance measurements provide a clear view on the development of gastric strain into a rumination episode. On impedance a rumination episode will present itself as a reflux episode, occurring closely after/before gastric straining observed on manometry.

Treatment

Previous studies suggest that the rumination syndrome is a learned behavior caused by gastrointestinal discomfort, as well as a reaction to stressful life events.[1,16,17] Treatment of the rumination syndrome is currently based on behavioral breathing therapy or cognitive therapy with biofeedback.[9,19] Both treatments are believed to compete with the urge to regurgitate and have yielded positive outcomes in previous studies.[9,17,20] Current advancements in physiology measurements have made it possible to better identify the rumination syndrome. In theory, each variation of the rumination syndrome could be treated according to the specific mechanism and triggers. For example, one study concluded that supragastric belching responds favorably to behavioral therapy

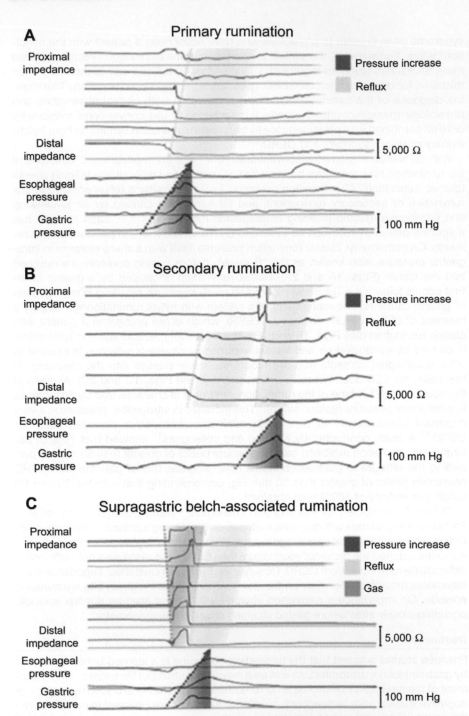

Fig. 1. Rumination variants as measured by combined ambulatory manometry and pH-impedance monitoring. (*A*) Primary rumination, (*B*) secondary rumination, (*C*) supragastric belch–associated rumination. (*From* Kessing BF, Bredenoord AJ, Smout AJ. Objective manometric criteria for the rumination syndrome. Am J Gastroenterol 2014;109:58; with permission from Macmillan Publishers Ltd.)

performed by a speech therapist.[21] The latter suggests that patients who exhibit supragastric rumination would also benefit from behavioral therapy.[17] However, secondary rumination appears to be triggered by reflux episodes, which in theory could benefit more from treatment of the reflux disease, because patients will ruminate only when they sense reflux episodes.[17] Based on this idea, proton pump inhibitor could also reduce the number of rumination episodes by decreasing the severity of heartburn.[17] However, in most cases, rumination will still occur, because weakly acidic reflux can also trigger rumination episodes.[17]

BELCHING DISORDERS
Pathophysiology

Belching is the audible escape of air from the esophagus into the pharynx. There are 2 types of belches: the so-called gastric belch and the supragastric belch.[4] Gastric belching is the escape of swallowed intragastric air that enters the esophagus during TLESR.[22] TLESRs are triggered by distension of the proximal stomach and allow venting of air from the stomach, thereby serving as a gastric decompression mechanism and preventing passage of large volumes of gas through the pylorus into the intestines. TLESRs are therefore referred to as the belch reflex.[23,24] Subsequently, esophageal distension caused by the refluxed air leads to relaxation of the UES, through which the air can escape from the esophagus.[25,26] Gastric belches usually occur 25 to 30 times per day and are physiologic. Gastric belches are involuntary and are controlled entirely by reflexes.[27]

In supragastric belches, the air does not originate from the stomach but is ingested immediately before it is expelled again. This phenomenon is most often caused by a contraction of the diaphragm, which creates a negative pressure in the thoracic cavity and the esophagus. Subsequent relaxation of the UES results in inflow of air into the esophagus. The air is suctioned into the esophagus and immediately expelled again in pharyngeal direction using straining (**Fig. 3**).[4,28] A second mechanism exists in which the air is injected into the esophagus through contraction of pharyngeal muscles; this mechanism is more rarely used.

Supragastric belches are seen in some patients as a behavioral response to abdominal pain or discomfort.[3] However, the cause of supragastric belching observed as an isolated disorder is still unknown. Some studies suggest that psychological factors, such as anxiety and stress, may play an important role.[3]

Clinical Evaluation and Diagnostic Approach

Diagnosis of belching disorders is based on the clinical history and the typical pattern on pH-impedance monitoring. HRM can be useful to identify the exact mechanism of supragastric belching but is not required. Some patients present themselves with isolated frequent belching, which may reach up to 20 times a minute.[3] These patients often show spells of excessive belching during their consultation. Many patients stop belching during speaking and it has been shown that patients belch less when distracted.[29] Furthermore, supragastric belching is never observed during sleep.[30] Patients with excessive isolated supragastric belching usually have no other symptoms besides, at times, dyspeptic symptoms.[3] The presence of weight loss, pain, dysphagia, heartburn, and regurgitation is an indication for further diagnostic evaluation. Usually, history is enough to establish a diagnosis but sometimes impedance monitoring is required to distinguish excessive supragastric belching from GERD and rumination.[11] With combined HRM and pH impedance, the typical mechanisms of supragastric belches can be identified. Because of a contraction of the diaphragm, the esophagogastric junction moves distally and a decrease in pressure in the esophagus is observed. Subsequently, HRM shows relaxation of the UES.[3] During impedance, a supragastric belch is observed as an increase in impedance (when the UES opens), starting in the proximal channel, and progressing to a distal channel, followed by a return to baseline starting in the distal channel (see **Fig. 3**). The diagnosis is made

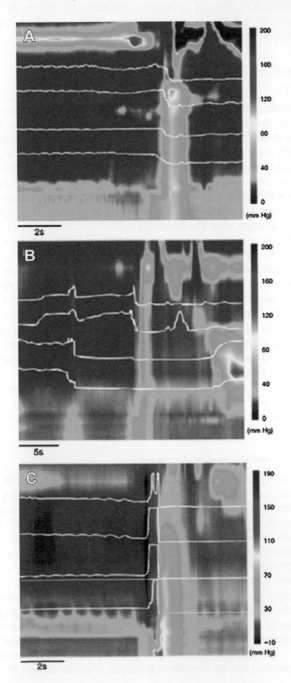

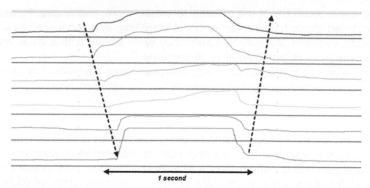

Fig. 3. Supragastric belch on pH-impedance measurement. The increase in impedance starts in the proximal channel (Z1) and the decrease in impedance starts in the distal channel (Z6), creating a V-shaped pattern.

when spells of supragastric belches are observed. As seen in **Fig. 3**, the LES remains closed and the UES opens repeatedly as air is sucked in and expelled rapidly.

It is important to point out that supragastric belching is not equivalent to air swallowing or aerophagia. Air swallowing is characterized by the act of swallowing of a certain volume of air, which is transported by the following peristaltic contraction to the stomach.[27,31] Peristaltic contractions are not seen during supragastric belching and do not form part of the mechanism of air ingestion in that disorder. In aerophagia, there is a real increase in ingested air, as a result of air swallowing, and is therefore distinct from excessive supragastric belching.[6]

Treatment

Patients presenting with isolated excessive supragastric belches often suffer from a decreased health-related quality of life.[32] Thus, it is important to take the symptoms seriously and try to treat these patients accordingly.[3] However, besides anecdotal reports there is still little evidence on treatment of patients with supragastric belching. There is only one open-label study, conducted by Hemmink and colleagues,[21] that provides some insight in the treatment of supragastric belching. In this study, behavioral therapy performed by a speech therapist was used. The therapy focused on

---

Fig. 2. The rumination variants as measured by combined HRM and pH-impedance monitoring. (*A*) Primary rumination: an increase in gastric pressure is followed by the flow of gastric content. Peak gastric pressure is observed during the flow of gastric content. Pressure in the esophageal lumen increases during the retrograde flow of gastric content and subsequent relaxation of the UES is observed. (*B*) Secondary rumination: similar to primary rumination but preceded by a spontaneous gastroesophageal reflux event. (*C*) Supragastric belch–associated rumination: initially, a movement of the diaphragm in aboral direction and a subatmospheric pressure in the esophageal lumen is observed. Relaxation of the UES is observed during the onset of inflow of air. The inflow of air is indicated by an antegrade increase in impedance. Thereafter, the esophageal air is immediately expulsed during which an increase in gastric pressure is observed. Subsequent flow of gastric content into the esophagus is observed during the increase in gastric pressure. The latter can be observed as a drop in impedance from baseline immediately after the supragastric belch. (*From* Kessing BF, Bredenoord AJ, Smout AJ. Objective manometric criteria for the rumination syndrome. Am J Gastroenterol 2014;109:55; with permission from Macmillan Publishers Ltd.)

explaining the mechanism of the disease to create more awareness. Furthermore, therapy included glottis training, conventional breathing, and vocal exercises.[21] During this study, symptom intensity and frequency were scored with a visual analogue scale. Both parameters improved after 10 sessions.[21]

Speech therapy thus seems promising; however, more evidence and research is needed to improve management of excessive supragastric belching.[21]

SUMMARY

Rumination and excessive supragastric belching are both an abnormal behavioral reaction, either as a response to abdominal pain or discomfort or spontaneous and psychological comorbidity often plays a role. Both disorders may present indistinguishable at first from other much more prevalent diseases, such as GERD. As a result, rumination and excessive supragastric belching are often misdiagnosed. Because of the low incidence of rumination and excessive belching disorder many physicians do not recognize these disorders. Therefore, physicians should be well informed regarding not only the clinical presentation but also the tools to facilitate the diagnosis. Recent evidence clearly demonstrates that diagnosis is easily made with manometry (HRM/conventional) combined with pH impedance. Moreover, with manometry and pH impedance we are able to, analyze the different underlying mechanisms that explain the clinical presentation and specify the management of the rumination variations and excessive supragastric belching.

In conclusion, rumination and excessive supragastric belching are increasingly recognized disorders, occurring also in otherwise healthy adults. By using manometry and pH-impedance monitoring it is possible to make an objective diagnosis of the rumination syndrome and belching disorders.

REFERENCES

1. Tucker E, Knowles K, Wright J, et al. Rumination variations: aetiology and classification of abnormal behavioural resposnses to digestive symptoms based on high-resolution manometry studies. Aliment Pharmacol Ther 2013;37:263–74.
2. Malcolm A, Thumshirn MB, Camilleri M, et al. Rumination syndrome. Mayo clin Proc 1997;72:646–52.
3. Bredenoord AJ. Management of belching, hiccups, and aerophagia. Clin Gastroenterol 2013;11:6–12.
4. Bredenoord AJ, Weusten BL, Sifrim D, et al. Aerophagia, gastric, and supragastric belching: a study using intraluminal electrical impedance monitoring. Gut 2004;53:1561–5.
5. Tack J, Talley NJ. Gastroduodenal disorder. Am J Gastroenterol 2010;105(4): 757–63.
6. Tack J, Talley NJ, Camilleri M, et al. Functional gastroduodenal disorders. Gastroenterology 2006;130(5):1466–79.
7. Rome Foundation. Guidelines—Rome III diagnostic criteria for functional gastrointestinal disorders. J Gastrointestin Liver Dis 2006;15(3):307–12.
8. O'brien MD, Bruce BK, Camilleri M. The rumination syndrome: clinical features rather than manometric diagnosis. Gastroenterology 1995;108(4):1024–9.
9. Tack J, Blondeau K, Boecxstaens V, et al. Review article: the pathophysiology, differential diagnosis and management of rumination syndrome. Aliment Pharmacol Ther 2011;33:782–8.
10. Longstreth GF, Thompson WG, Chey WD, et al. Functional bowel disorders. Gastroenterology 2006;130:1480–91.

11. Rommel N, Tack J, Arts J, et al. Rumination or belching-regurgitation? Differential diagnosis using oesophageal impedance-manometry. Neurogastroenterol Motil 2010;22:e97–104.

12. Tutuian R, Castell DO. Rumination documented by using combined multichannel intraluminal impedance and manometry. Clin Gastroenterol Hepatol 2004;2(4): 340–3.

13. Kessing BF, Govaert F, Masclee AA, et al. Impedance measurements and high-resolution manometry help to better define rumination episodes. Scand J Gastroenterol 2011;46(11):1310–5.

14. Thumshirn M, Camilleri M, Hanson RB, et al. Gastric mechanosensory and lower esophageal function in rumination syndrome. Am J Physiol 1998;275:G314–21.

15. Smout AJ, Breumelhof R. Voluntary induction of transient lower esophageal sphincter relaxations in an adult patient with the rumination syndrome. Am J Gastroenterol 1990;85:1621–5.

16. Chial HJ, Camilleri M, Williams DE, et al. Rumination syndrome in children and adolescents: diagnosis, treatment, and prognosis. Pediatrics 2003;111:158–62.

17. Kessing BF, Bredenoord AJ, Smout AJ. Objective manometric criteria for the rumination syndrome. Am J Gastroenterol 2014;109:52–9.

18. Weusten BL, Smout AJ. The secondary rumination syndrome. Eur J Gastroenterol Hepatol 1994;6:1171–6.

19. Khan S, Hyman PE, Oclin J, et al. Rumination syndrome in adolescents. J Pediatr 2000;136(4):528–31.

20. Chitkara DK, Van Tilburg M, Whitehead WE, et al. Teaching diaphrag- matic breathing for rumination syndrome. Am J Gastroenterol 2006;101:2449–52.

21. Hemmink GJ, Ten Cate L, Bredenoord AJ, et al. Speech therapy in patients with excessive supragastric belching—a pilot study. Neurogastroenterol Motil 2010; 22:24–8, e2–3.

22. Wyman JB, Dent J, Heddle R, et al. Control of belching by the lower esophageal sphincter. Gut 2004;53:1561–5.

23. Mittal RK, Rochester DF, McCallum RW. Electrical and mechanical activity in the human lower esophageal sphincter during diaphragmatic contraction. J Clin Invest 1988;81:1182–9.

24. Kessing BF, Conchillo JM, Bredenoord AJ, et al. Review article: the clinical relevance of transient lower esophageal pshincter relaxations in gastro-oesophageal reflux disease. Aliment Pharmacol Ther 2011;33:650–61.

25. Shaker R, Ren J, Kern M, et al. Mechanisms of airway protection and upper esophageal pshincter opening during belching. Am J Physiol 1992;262:G621–8.

26. Kahrilas PJ, Dodds WJ, Dent J, et al. Upper esophageal sphincter function during belching. Gastroenterology 1986;91:133–40.

27. Bredenoord AJ, Weusten BL, Timmer R, et al. Relationships between air swallowing, intragastric air, belching and gastro-oesophageal reflux. Neurogastroenterol Motil 2005;17:341–7.

28. Kessing BF, Bredenoord AJ, Smout AJ. Gastric belching and supragastric belching are two distinct pathophysiological entities: a study using combined high-resolution manometry and impedance monitoring. Gastroenterology 2012; 142:282.

29. Bredenoord AJ, Weusten BL, Timmer R, et al. Psychological factors affect the frequency of belching in patients with aerophagia. Am J Gastroenterol 2006;101: 2777–81.

30. Karamanolis G, Triantafyllou K, Tsiamoulos Z, et al. Effect of sleep on excessive belching: a 24-hour impedance-pH study. J Clin Gastroenterol 2010;44:332–4.

31. Pouderoux P, Ergun Ga, Lin S, et al. Esophageal bolus transit imaged by ultrafast computerized tomography. Gastroenterology 2006;130:1466–79.
32. Bredenoord AJ, Smout AJ. Impaired health-related quality of life in patients with excessive supragastric belching. Eur J Gastroenterol Hepatol 2010;22: 1420–3.

Uses of Esophageal Function Testing: Dysphagia

Etsuro Yazaki, PhD, MAGIP[a,b], Philip Woodland, MBBS, PhD[a,b], Daniel Sifrim, MD, PhD[a,b],*

KEYWORDS

- Dysphagia • Esophageal motility • High-resolution manometry
- Impedance planimetry

KEY POINTS

- Esophageal function testing should be used for differential diagnosis of dysphagia after exclusion of structural causes.
- High-resolution manometry increases diagnostic yield and can predict treatment outcomes in achalasia.
- Impedance planimetry can help to identify abnormalities in esophagogastric junction distensibility in achalasia and eosinophilic esophagitis.

INTRODUCTION

Dysphagia is defined as a difficulty (or a sensation of difficulty) of food passage, which may be difficult with initiating a swallow (oropharyngeal dysphagia) or the sensation that foods and/or liquids are hindered in their passage from the mouth to the stomach (esophageal dysphagia).[1] This distinction can be made from a careful medical history (oropharyngeal vs esophageal) in about 80% to 85% of cases.[2] This article discusses the use of esophageal function testing in the context of esophageal dysphagia.

Esophageal dysphagia may have structural/obstructive causes, secondary to motility disorders, or may be predominantly sensory. In a patient presenting with dysphagia the priority is to exclude a structural cause such as an esophageal malignancy. Hence, if the history is suggestive, the first clinical assessments for dysphagia should be endoscopy and/or barium swallow. At endoscopy, eosinophilic esophagitis can also be diagnosed or excluded by way of esophageal biopsy. **Box 1** summarizes common causes of dysphagia that should be excluded before esophageal function testing. There are other rare causes of structural esophageal dysphagia such as lymphocytic esophagitis, esophageal compression by cardiovascular abnormalities, or

[a] Centre for Digestive Diseases, Barts and The London School of Medicine and Dentistry, Queen Mary University of London, London, UK; [b] Gastrointestinal Physiology Unit, Barts Health NHS Trust, Royal London Hospital, London, UK
* Corresponding author. Wingate Institute of Neurogastroenterology, 26 Ashfield Street, London E12AJ, United Kingdom.
E-mail address: d.sifrim@qmul.ac.uk

Gastrointest Endoscopy Clin N Am 24 (2014) 643–654
http://dx.doi.org/10.1016/j.giec.2014.06.008
1052-5157/14/$ – see front matter © 2014 Elsevier Inc. All rights reserved.

> **Box 1**
> **Causes of dysphagia that should be excluded before esophageal function testing**
>
> Tumors (esophageal, lung, lymphoma)
>
> Vascular compression (aortic, auricular)
>
> Esophageal rings and webs
>
> Chemical or radiation injury
>
> Peptic stricture
>
> Infectious esophagitis (herpes virus, *Candida albicans*)
>
> Eosinophilic esophagitis

esophageal involvement of Crohn disease, which can be considered if medical history is suggestive.

After exclusion of structural causes for dysphagia, esophageal function testing is used to assess motility disorders. Dysphagia can be the consequence of hypermotility or hypomotility of the circular and/or longitudinal muscle layers of the esophagus. It has recently been shown that decreased esophageal or esophagogastric junction (EGJ) distensibility can provoke dysphagia. The most well-established esophageal dysmotility is achalasia. Other motility disorders, including diffuse esophageal spasm, hypercontractile esophagus, and severe hypomotility can also cause dysphagia.[3] High-resolution manometry (HRM) is currently regarded as the gold standard investigation to identify and classify esophageal motility disorders. Simultaneous measurement of HRM and intraluminal impedance (high-resolution impedance manometry [HRIM]) can be useful to assess both motility and bolus transit.[4] Impedance planimetry (EndoFlip) has recently been introduced to measure distensibility of the esophageal body and EGJ in patients with achalasia and eosinophilic esophagitis.[5,6] This article discusses the use of esophageal function testing in patients with esophageal dysphagia after exclusion of structural abnormalities by normal endoscopy and or radiological examination.

DYSPHAGIA ASSOCIATED WITH ESOPHAGEAL MOTILITY DISORDERS DEFINED IN THE CHICAGO CLASSIFICATION
Achalasia

The most established esophageal dysmotility is achalasia. At endoscopy, achalasia can be suggested by esophageal food residue, appearance of esophageal body, and tightness of the lower esophageal sphincter (LES). HRM should be used to confirm diagnosis of achalasia and to identify the subtype of achalasia.

The Chicago Classification criteria of esophageal motility disorders are currently the standard reference for HRM classification.[7] According to this classification, 3 achalasia subtypes (shown in **Fig. 1**) are defined. As expected in achalasia, each is characterized by a failed relaxation of the lower esophageal sphincter during swallows (as determined on HRM by an LES integrated relaxation pressure [IRP], of >15 mm Hg), and by an absence of ordered peristalsis. In type I (classic) achalasia the IRP greater than or equal to 15 mm Hg is associated with a complete absence of esophageal pressure: 100% failed peristalsis. In type II (achalasia with esophageal compression) there is an IRP greater than or equal to 15 mm Hg and at least 20% of wet swallows associated with columns of panesophageal pressurization with greater than 30 mm Hg Type III (spastic achalasia) is defined as an IRP greater than or equal to 15 mm Hg with at least

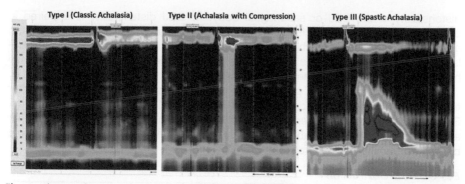

Fig. 1. Three subtypes of achalasia defined by HRM. Type II is considered the phenotype with best prognosis.

20% of wet swallows associated with either a preserved fragment of distal peristalsis or a premature (spastic, distal latency <4.5 seconds) contraction.[7]

As well as providing an excellent means of diagnosis, HRM can help predict outcome and guide choice of clinical intervention in achalasia. It has been shown that type II achalasia has the best outcome to treatment, followed by type I, then type III.[8] A study by Boeckxstaens and colleagues[9] showed that for type II and I achalasia outcomes were similar for pneumatic dilatation and surgical myotomy (although young men tend to do better with myotomy). In type III achalasia, outcomes are better with myotomy. Data regarding subtype outcomes from peroral endoscopic myotomy (POEM) are awaited.

Persistent Dysphagia After Treatment in Achalasia

A significant group of patients with achalasia present with recurrent dysphagia months or several years after successful initial treatment. It is common to perform esophageal function testing on these patients. The most useful tests in this situation (again, after excluding a structural cause) are HRM and a timed barium esophagram. Perhaps the most important question is whether there is residual increased pressure at the EGJ. Patients may have persistent increased resistance at the EGJ either because of increased residual EGJ pressures or decreased distensibility resulting in bolus retention. It is expected that peristaltic activity is still not present. The timed barium esophagogram (TBE) is a simple fluoroscopic evaluation of bolus clearance of esophagus, and is often a useful adjunct to HRM.[10] It involves taking multiple sequential films at predefined time intervals after swallowing a fixed volume of a barium solution of a specific density. After swallowing, upright radiographs are usually taken at 1, 3, and 5 minutes to assess barium clearance.

The patient with dysphagia after treatment of achalasia with a moderate to high IRP and a retained barium column on TBE requires retreatment. Barium column stasis on TBE predicts recurrent symptoms in patients with long-standing achalasia.[11]

Esophageal impedance can also give an idea of the level of liquid retention. Cho and colleagues[12] recently reported an excellent agreement between TBE and HRIM for assessing bolus retention at 5 minutes. As more data and confidence in the technique are gained it is possible that HRIM will be used as a single test to assess bolus retention and motor function in the management of treated achalasia.

The functional lumen imaging probe (EndoFLIP) uses impedance planimetry to calculate luminal diameters and, together with intraluminal pressure measurements, can be used to calculate distensibiltiy.[13] EndoFLIP has been used to measure distensibility of the EGJ or esophageal body.[6,14] EGJ distensibility is impaired in patients with achalasia, and is associated with the degree of esophageal emptying and clinical response. As such, it can be used to evaluate treatment efficacy in achalasia.[15] At present, impedance planimetry is only available in a few centers, but it may have the potential to guide therapy in the future if outcome studies are performed.

In summary, evaluation of patients with achalasia and recurrent symptoms after treatment can be widely performed using TBE and HRM with or without impedance. Symptomatic patients with persistent retention on TBE should be retreated. Whether asymptomatic patients with abnormal TBE, detected during routine follow-up, should be treated remains controversial.

EGJ Outflow Obstruction

Some patients with dysphagia without initial endoscopic or radiologic evidence of structural obstruction display increased IRP (as in achalasia) and normal peristalsis (therefore excluding a diagnosis of achalasia) during HRM. This pattern is classified as EGJ outflow obstruction.[7] A study reported that among 1000 consecutive HRM studies, 16 patients fulfilled the criteria characterized by impaired EGJ relaxation, often accompanied by increased intrabolus pressure, and intact peristalsis.[16]

In some patients the cause of EGJ outflow obstruction is mechanical obstruction (**Box 2**). It is recommended that patients with this motility pattern have endoscopic examination (if not already performed) and computed tomography (CT) or endoscopic ultrasonography evaluation of the EGJ. Note that patients with hiatal hernias are within this group because it has been shown that sliding hiatus hernias alter the pressure dynamics through the EGJ.[17] Patients with an EGJ outflow obstruction after surgical fundoplication are discussed later.

In the remainder of patients the failed relaxation of the EGJ is not mechanical, and the nature of this phenotype is the subject of some debate. It has been postulated that it represents an incomplete expression of achalasia (although this has not yet been shown histopathologically).[18] If mechanical obstruction (including sliding hiatal hernia) is excluded, it is considered a reasonable approach to dilate as in achalasia (although myotomy is less often practiced in this scenario).

Distal Esophageal Spasm

Distal esophageal spasm (DES) is an uncommon motility disorder often associated with dysphagia. As technology has evolved, so has the definition of esophageal spasm. With conventional manometry the diagnosis was defined by the presence of simultaneous contractions as well as preserved peristalsis, and was called diffuse esophageal spasm.[19] The greater resolution of HRM has led to a definition that takes into account

---

Box 2
Mechanical causes of EGJ outflow obstruction

EGJ mucosal/submucosal neoplasm

Fibrotic stenosis (eg, after inflammation/radiotherapy)

Eosinophilic esophagitis

Obstructing esophageal varices

Sliding hiatus hernia

After fundoplication[a]

[a] Postsurgical obstruction is not covered by the Chicago Classification.

the absence of adequate peristaltic inhibition. The key to the diagnosis is now measurement of the distal latency (the time between onset of the swallow and the deceleration point of the esophageal contraction, which cannot be measured on conventional manometry). The Chicago Classification diagnostic criteria for DES include a normal IRP and greater than or equal to 20% premature contractions (ie, distal latency <4.5 seconds).[7]

The difference between DES and type III achalasia is in the adequate or inadequate relaxation of the EGJ. In achalasia there can be significant esophageal shortening leading to pseudorelaxation of the EGJ. HRM does not have this limitation, and is therefore the investigation of choice in making this diagnostic distinction (**Fig. 2**).

If symptoms of pain or dysphagia are associated with DES then treatment is indicated. First it is sensible to rule out gastroesophageal reflux with reflux testing or empirical proton pump inhibitor treatment because DES and reflux frequently coexist (although the pathophysiologic relationship is not well defined). Other medical therapies are designed to relax smooth muscle or overcome the defective inhibitory neural function. Smooth muscle relaxants such as nitrates[20] and calcium channel antagonists[21] are often used, but controlled trials are lacking. The phosphodiesterase-5 inhibitor sildenafil blocks degradation of NO, resulting in a more prolonged smooth muscle relaxation and seems effective in relieving symptoms and improving manometric findings in spasm.[22] In addition, endoscopically injected botulinum toxin has been shown to have some benefit in terms of pain and dysphagia.[23] A future possibility for therapy is POEM, in which a long proximal myotomy has theoretic potential. There are preliminary reports suggesting some benefit.[24]

Hypercontractile Esophagus

Hypercontractile esophagus or hypertensive esophageal peristalsis used to refer to so-called nutcracker esophagus using conventional manometry.[19] The clinical relevance of nutcracker esophagus seems variable because its presence may or may not be associated with dysphagia. Tutuian and Castell[4] reported that 97% of patients with nutcracker esophagus had complete bolus transit assessed by combined multichannel intraluminal impedance and manometry. In the Chicago Classification, the distal contractile integral (DCI; an integral that takes into account the amplitude, length, and duration of contraction) is used to diagnose nutcracker esophagus, in which a

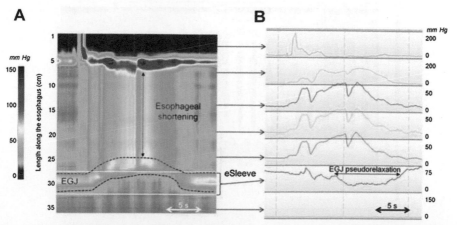

Fig. 2. Esophageal shortening observed using HRM (*A*) can cause pseudorelaxation of EGJ on conventional manometry (*B*). (*From* Roman S, Kahrilas P. Distal esophageal spasm. Dysphagia 2012;27:115–23; with permission.)

mean value of 5000 to 8000 mm Hg/s/cm is found. The classification also now defines hypercontractile esophagus, in which at least 1 wet-swallow DCI is greater than 8000 mm Hg·s·cm (a value not seen in any asymptomatic individual) with single or multiple peaks (jackhammer esophagus) in a context of normal EGJ relaxation.[7] Hypercontractile esophagus can be associated with dysphagia or chest pain.[25] Jackhammer esophagus (**Fig. 3**) is most likely to be accompanied by dysphagia.[26] Hypercontractility can be secondary to other underlying disorders such as EGJ outflow obstruction, so it is important to ensure that the IRP is normal before making the diagnosis. Treatment options are largely as described earlier for spasm.

Esophageal Hypomotility

One of the important roles of esophageal function testing is to evaluate unexplained dysphagia. Esophageal dysmotility patterns described so far are of major motor disorders associated with dysphagia. With the introduction of HRM, more detailed assessment of peristaltic integrity became possible, which brought the new manometric classifications of esophageal hypomotility (ie, weak peristalsis with small/large peristaltic defects or frequent failed peristalsis).[7]

At the extreme of esophageal hypomotility, HRM findings of 100% failed peristalsis with normal EGJ relaxation is defined as absent peristalsis.[7] Symptoms can be dysphagia and/or gastroesophageal reflux, and absent peristalsis can be a presentation of esophageal involvement in connective tissue disease (scleroderma; **Fig. 4**), which should be actively investigated.

Lesser degrees of esophageal hypomotility can be associated with dysphagia (although less reliably) and failure of esophageal bolus transit. Roman and colleagues[27] reported that weak peristalsis, but not failed peristalsis, occurred significantly more frequently in patients with unexplained dysphagia than in control subjects. The clinical relevance of esophageal hypomotility (particularly with small peristaltic defects) is not clear, especially because not all patients with weak peristalsis complain of dysphagia. Evaluation of bolus transit may give a clearer indication of clinical relevance. Kahrilas and colleagues[28] reported that incomplete bolus transit frequently occurred in the distal esophagus when contraction amplitude was less than 20 mm Hg. Esophageal pressure topography plots with breaks greater than 5 cm in

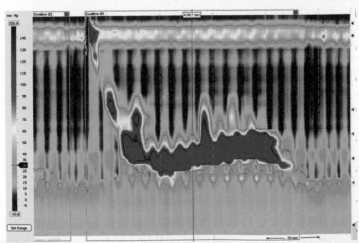

Fig. 3. Jackhammer esophagus: this type of hypermotility can be associated with dysphagia and/or chest pain.

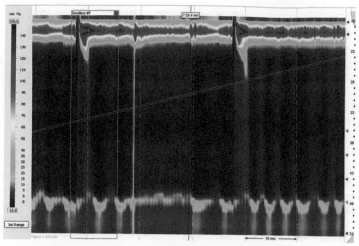

Fig. 4. Absent peristalsis in a patient with confirmed scleroderma.

20 mm Hg isobaric contour were closely associated with incomplete bolus transit.[27] HRIM is useful to investigate this patient group by measuring esophageal motility and bolus transport simultaneously.[4,27] Using impedance channels, it is possible to evaluate whether hypomotility is associated with incomplete bolus transit, and whether this corresponds with symptoms of dysphagia. A common treatment approach to patients with hypomotility and dysphagia is to use prokinetic therapy. Motilin agonists such as erythromycin, and dopamine antagonists such as metoclopramide, have been used, but a clinical benefit is not established.

INVESTIGATION OF DYSPHAGIA RESULTING FROM OTHER CAUSES
Dysphagia with Normal Esophageal Peristalsis on Wet Swallows

There is a patient group with dysphagia, especially with intermittent dysphagia for solids, whose HRM seems to be normal using the Chicago Classification. The limitation of diagnostic yield at HRM is that normal values are obtained from 10 wet swallows of 5 mL of water. Provocative swallows such as larger volume of water or solid swallowing at HRM might reproduce dysphagia in such a patient group and increase a diagnostic yield.

Sweis and colleagues[29,30] described use of standardized solid food and showed that abnormal pressure events at HRM were associated with dysphagia. **Fig. 5** shows

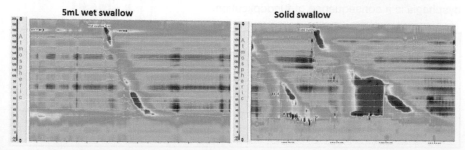

Fig. 5. This patient presented with dysphagia and chest pain during meals. Peristalsis was weak during liquid swallows (*left*). However, bread swallows (*right*) induced esophageal segmental pressurization associated with typical symptoms.

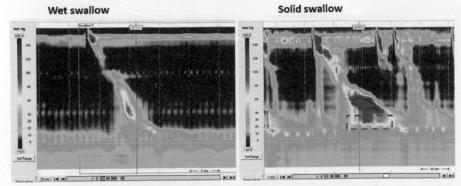

Wet swallow   **Solid swallow**

Fig. 6. This patient presented with dysphagia after Nissen fundoplication. Peristalsis and IRP were normal during wet swallows (*left*). However, bread swallows (*right*) induced esophageal segmental pressurization within the double high-pressure zone (*dotted area*) associated with typical symptoms.

an example of solid swallowing for one of our patients with solid dysphagia with and without retrosternal pain/pressure. Use of solid swallowing at HRM may be a helpful provocative test to diagnose abnormal pressure events not produced with standard 5-mL wet swallows. A standard classification is lacking, but it may be useful when careful consideration is given to the association of pressure events and symptoms.

Dysphagia Following Antireflux Surgery

Dysphagia is a recognized complication of fundoplication, and patients with dysphagia after antireflux surgery are often evaluated by HRM. In contrast with the preoperative state, normal values of the IRP are not described after antireflux surgery. A high IRP (in association with a high intrabolus pressure) may be a sign of EGJ outflow obstruction secondary to a too-tight fundoplication. Recent studies using HRM have reported that a dual high-pressure zone (HPZ) at the EGJ is a sign of failed or disrupted fundoplication.[31] The dual HPZ is caused by either slipped wrap or intrathoracic fundoplication.

A small series of postfundoplication patients with dysphagia and a double HPZ were studied with HRM at our unit. IRP did not reveal abnormal EGJ dynamics on wet swallows, and rapid swallow provocation tests provoked no obvious changes in pressure tomography at EGJ. An increased pressure within the dual HPZ during solid swallows was the only significant change and this could be an objective parameter to assess postfundoplication patients with dysphagia (**Fig. 6**). **Table 1** summarizes our preliminary findings. Redo fundoplication and dilatation are therapeutic options when dysphagia is a consequence of fundoplication.

Table 1 IRP and pressure within dual high-pressure zone (DHPZ) during different types of swallows		
	IRP (mm Hg)	**Pressure in DHPZ (mm Hg)**
WS	8.65 ± 6.17	7.01 ± 4.42
MRS	5.75 ± 5.15	7.12 ± 5.96
200RS	4.62 ± 4.56	6.17 ± 7.75
SS	10.12 ± 2.92	25.41 ± 17.87[a]

[a] P = .003 against WS.
Abbreviations: MRS, multiple rapid swallows; WS, wet swallows; SS, solid swallows; 200RS, 200ml rapid swallows.

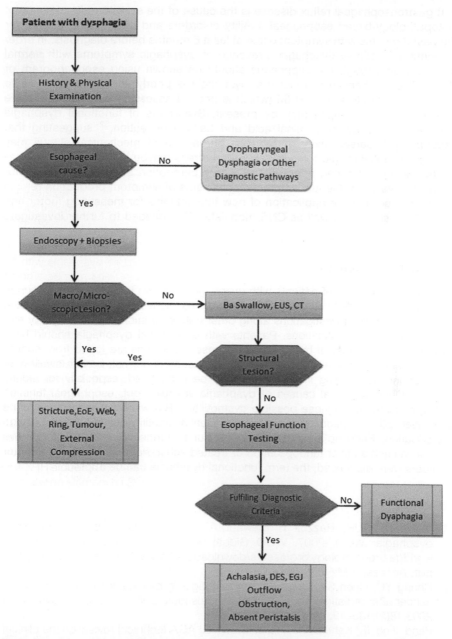

Fig. 7. Diagnosis and management of esophageal dysphagia. EoE, eosinophilic esophagitis; EUS, endoscopic ultrasonography.

Functional Dysphagia

Patients with dysphagia without any abnormalities at endoscopy or esophageal function testing can be classified as functional dysphagia. The Rome III diagnostic criteria for functional dysphagia are (1) a sense of solid and/or liquid food sticking, lodging, or passing abnormally through the esophagus; (2) absence of evidence that gastroesophageal reflux disease is the cause of the symptom; (3) absence of histopathology-based esophageal motility disorders and all 3 criteria fulfilled for the past 3 months with symptom onset at least 6 months before diagnosis. In order to confirm functional dysphagia, presence of dysphagic symptoms with normal bolus transit through the esophagus should be shown using esophagogram or HRIM. The mechanism of functional dysphagia is poorly understood. Peristaltic dysfunction not elicited by HRM (which is poor at assessing longitudinal muscle contraction, for example) may be present. Symptoms of functional dysphagia can be induced by intraluminal acid and balloon distention,[32] suggesting that esophageal hypersensitivity or reduced perception of mechanical stimuli may have a pathophysiologic role. Psychological stress maybe important in some patients, because this can affect both sensory perception and esophageal motor function.[33] As such, the fundamental mechanisms of symptom production remain poorly defined. Further application of new technologies for measuring motor and sensory physiology as well as CNS modulation[34] is needed to further investigate this condition.

DIAGNOSTIC FLOWCHART

A diagnostic flowchart of patients with dysphagia is shown in **Fig. 7**. First, accurate medical history needs to be taken. When symptoms suggest a nonesophageal cause, the patient requires investigations along other pathways such as neurologic or ear, nose, and throat investigations. Patients with esophageal dysphagia should have endoscopy with biopsy. If macroscopic/microscopic lesions are found from endoscopy, patients are treated accordingly. If endoscopy is normal, barium swallow or other diagnostic imaging investigations can be considered, especially for elderly patients. Once structural causes of dysphagia are ruled out, esophageal function testing is useful to diagnose possible dysmotility. HRM with or without impedance is an ideal option to diagnose primary esophageal dysmotility defined by the Chicago Classification. EndoFlip or TBE can be useful to further evaluate postoperative dysphagia such as after fundoplication or treated achalasia. If no esophageal motor disorders were diagnosed, the term functional dysphagia can be applied.

REFERENCES

1. Malagelada JR, Bazzoli F, Elewaut A, et al. WGO practice guideline - dysphagia: WGO. 2007. WGO Global Guideline. Available at: http://www.worldgastroenterology.org/assets/downloads/en/pdf/guidelines/08_dysphagia.pdf. Accessed May 23, 2014.
2. Chang YC, Chen SY, Lui LT, et al. Dysphagia in patients with nasopharyngeal cancer after radiation therapy: a videofluoroscopic swallowing study. Dysphagia 2003;18(2):135–43.
3. Pandolfino JE, Kahrilas PJ, Association AG. AGA technical review on the clinical use of esophageal manometry. Gastroenterology 2005;128(1):209–24.
4. Tutuian R, Castell DO. Combined multichannel intraluminal impedance and manometry clarifies esophageal function abnormalities: study in 350 patients. Am J Gastroenterol 2004;99(6):1011–9.
5. Massey BT. EndoFLIP assessment of achalasia therapy: interpreting the distensibility data is a bit of a stretch. Gastroenterology 2013;144(4):e17–8.
6. Kwiatek MA, Hirano I, Kahrilas PJ, et al. Mechanical properties of the esophagus in eosinophilic esophagitis. Gastroenterology 2011;140(1):82–90.

7. Bredenoord AJ, Fox M, Kahrilas PJ, et al. Chicago classification criteria of esophageal motility disorders defined in high resolution esophageal pressure topography. Neurogastroenterol Motil 2012;24(Suppl 1):57–65.

8. Pandolfino JE, Kwiatek MA, Nealis T. Achalasia: a new clinically relevant classification by high-resolution manometry. Gastroenterology 2008;135(5): 1526–33.

9. Boeckxstaens GE, Annese V, des Varannes SB, et al. Pneumatic dilation versus laparoscopic Heller's myotomy for idiopathic achalasia. N Engl J Med 2011; 364(19):1807–16.

10. Kostic SV, Rice TW, Baker ME, et al. Timed barium esophagogram: a simple physiologic assessment for achalasia. J Thorac Cardiovasc Surg 2000;120(5): 935–43.

11. Rohof WO, Lei A, Boeckxstaens GE. Esophageal stasis on a timed barium esophagogram predicts recurrent symptoms in patients with long-standing achalasia. Am J Gastroenterol 2013;108(1):49–55.

12. Cho YK, Lipowska AM, Nicodème F, et al. Assessing bolus retention in achalasia using high-resolution manometry with impedance: a comparator study with timed barium esophagram. Am J Gastroenterol 2014;109(6):829–35.

13. McMahon BP, Frøkjaer JB, Kunwald P, et al. The functional lumen imaging probe (FLIP) for evaluation of the esophagogastric junction. Am J Physiol Gastrointest Liver Physiol 2007;292(1):G377–84.

14. Kwiatek MA, Pandolfino JE, Hirano I, et al. Esophagogastric junction distensibility assessed with an endoscopic functional luminal imaging probe (EndoFLIP). Gastrointest Endosc 2010;72(2):272–8.

15. Rohof WO, Hirsch DP, Kessing BF, et al. Efficacy of treatment for patients with achalasia depends on the distensibility of the esophagogastric junction. Gastroenterology 2012;143(2):328–35.

16. Scherer JR, Kwiatek MA, Soper NJ, et al. Functional esophagogastric junction obstruction with intact peristalsis: a heterogeneous syndrome sometimes akin to achalasia. J Gastrointest Surg 2009;13(12):2219–25.

17. Pandolfino JE, Kwiatek MA, Ho K, et al. Unique features of esophagogastric junction pressure topography in hiatus hernia patients with dysphagia. Surgery 2010; 147(1):57–64.

18. Roman S, Kahrilas PJ. Challenges in the swallowing mechanism: nonobstructive dysphagia in the era of high-resolution manometry and impedance. Gastroenterol Clin North Am 2011;40(4):823–35, ix–x.

19. Spechler SJ, Castell DO. Classification of oesophageal motility abnormalities. Gut 2001;49(1):145–51.

20. Swamy N. Esophageal spasm: clinical and manometric response to nitroglycerine and long acting nitrites. Gastroenterology 1977;72(1):23–7.

21. Baunack AR, Weihrauch TR. Clinical efficacy of nifedipine and other calcium antagonists in patients with primary esophageal motor dysfunctions. Arzneimittelforschung 1991;41(6):595–602.

22. Eherer AJ, Schwetz I, Hammer HF, et al. Effect of sildenafil on oesophageal motor function in healthy subjects and patients with oesophageal motor disorders. Gut 2002;50(6):758–64.

23. Storr M, Allescher HD, Rösch T, et al. Treatment of symptomatic diffuse esophageal spasm by endoscopic injection of botulinum toxin: a prospective study with long term follow-up. Gastrointest Endosc 2001;54(6):18A.

24. Minami H, Isomoto H, Yamaguchi N, et al. Peroral endoscopic myotomy (POEM) for diffuse esophageal spasm. Endoscopy 2014;46(Suppl 1 UCTN):E79–81.

25. Ghosh S, Pandolfino J, Rice J, et al. Impaired deglutitive EGJ relaxation in clinical esophageal manometry: a quantitative analysis of 400 patients and 75 controls. Am J Physiol Gastrointest Liver Physiol 2007;293(4):G878–85.
26. Roman S, Pandolfino JE, Chen J, et al. Phenotypes and clinical context of hypercontractility in high-resolution esophageal pressure topography (EPT). Am J Gastroenterol 2012;107(1):37–45.
27. Roman S, Lin Z, Kwiatek MA, et al. Weak peristalsis in esophageal pressure topography: classification and association with dysphagia. Am J Gastroenterol 2011;106(2):349–56.
28. Kahrilas P, Dodds W, Hogan W. Effect of peristaltic dysfunction on esophageal volume clearance. Gastroenterology 1988;94(1):73–80.
29. Sweis R, Anggiansah A, Wong T, et al. Normative values and inter-observer agreement for liquid and solid bolus swallows in upright and supine positions as assessed by esophageal high-resolution manometry. Neurogastroenterol Motil 2011;23(6):509.e198.
30. Sweis R, Anggiansah A, Wong T, et al. Assessment of esophageal dysfunction and symptoms during and after a standardized test meal: development and clinical validation of a new methodology utilizing high-resolution manometry. Neurogastroenterol Motil 2014;26(2):215–28.
31. Hoshino M, Srinivasan A, Mittal SK. High-resolution manometry patterns of lower esophageal sphincter complex in symptomatic post-fundoplication patients. J Gastrointest Surg 2012;16(4):705–14.
32. Deschner WK, Maher KA, Cattau EL, et al. Manometric responses to balloon distention in patients with nonobstructive dysphagia. Gastroenterology 1989; 97(5):1181–5.
33. Drossman DA, Corazziari E, Delvaux M, et al. ROME III: the functional gastrointestinal disorders. 3rd edition. Yale University Section of Digestive Disease. MacLean, VA: Degnon Associates; 2006.
34. Suntrup S, Teismann I, Wollbrink A, et al. Altered cortical swallowing processing in patients with functional dysphagia: a preliminary study. PLoS One 2014;9(2): e89665.

Diagnostic Work-Up of GERD

Marcelo F. Vela, MD, MSCR

KEYWORDS

- Gastroesophageal reflux disease (GERD) • Heartburn • Proton pump inhibitor test
- Endoscopy • pH monitoring • Impedance-pH monitoring

KEY POINTS

- Gastroesophageal reflux disease (GERD) may be diagnosed by symptoms and a positive PPI test in some settings; however, it is important to be aware of the limited sensitivity and specificity of this approach as a diagnostic intervention.
- The finding of erosive esophagitis on endoscopy provides robust evidence of GERD but endoscopy is normal in most patients with GERD.
- Ambulatory reflux monitoring is the gold standard for diagnosing GERD.
- In some patients without good response to PPI, the reported symptoms are due to non-GERD causes; a negative work up can exclude GERD and help direct the diagnostic and treatment efforts toward other causes.
- Work up of patients with PPI-refractory symptoms should proceed in this order: optimization of PPI therapy; investigation for non-GERD causes by endoscopy for typical symptoms as well as ears-nose-throat, allergy, and pulmonary evaluation for atypical presentations; and, finally, reflux monitoring if the reason for refractoriness remains unclear.

INTRODUCTION

Gastroesophageal reflux disease (GERD) is a very common clinical problem. Heartburn or acid regurgitation is experienced on a weekly basis by nearly 20% of the US population, with an annual prevalence of up to 59%.[1] GERD may be diagnosed by symptom assessment through patient history or GERD questionnaires, response to a trial of proton pump inhibitors (PPIs), findings of reflux-related esophageal mucosal damage by endoscopy, or by establishing the presence of pathologic reflux on prolonged ambulatory monitoring with pH or impedance-pH. In routine clinical practice, GERD is frequently diagnosed by symptom presentation along with a good response to a PPI trial. Although this constitutes a simple and reasonable approach in the appropriate setting (eg, primary care of uncomplicated patients), it is important to bear in mind its limitations.

In addition to careful history-taking for typical symptoms of GERD, validated questionnaires are available to measure specific symptoms and GERD-related quality of life

Division of Gastroenterology, Mayo Clinic Arizona, 13400 East Shea Boulevard, Scottsdale, AZ 85259, USA
E-mail address: Vela.Marcelo@mayo.edu

Gastrointest Endoscopy Clin N Am 24 (2014) 655–666
http://dx.doi.org/10.1016/j.giec.2014.07.002
1052-5157/14/$ – see front matter © 2014 Elsevier Inc. All rights reserved.

giendo.theclinics.com

scales. These instruments can be helpful but they generally have similar specificity and sensitivity compared with clinical examination by a gastroenterologist. Therefore, they are most commonly used in clinical trials.

Upper endoscopy is indicated for patients with alarm features such as dysphagia, bleeding, or weight loss, and in patients with typical symptoms that do not respond appropriately to PPI therapy. The finding of erosive esophagitis on endoscopy provides robust evidence of GERD, but this lesion is present in only one-third of untreated patients[2] and it is uncommon in those that are in treatment with a PPI. Random biopsies to document GERD in patients with normal endoscopy are not advised because of the limited diagnostic capabilities of conventional histology for this purpose.

When endoscopy is negative in patients with an uncertain diagnosis of GERD or a suboptimal response to PPI, further work up involves objective quantification of gastroesophageal reflux. This can be accomplished through pH monitoring (catheter-based or wireless), which can establish whether a pathologic amount of acid reflux is present and may provide insight regarding the association between reflux episodes and reported symptoms. Impedance-pH monitoring enables measurement of not only acid, but also nonacid (with a pH >4) reflux episodes. Nonacid reflux may be important in patients with PPI-refractory symptoms. Objective documentation of GERD by endoscopy or reflux monitoring is mandatory before antireflux surgery. Of note, barium esophagram and esophageal manometry cannot establish whether GERD is present and are not useful to diagnose it. However, these tests, especially manometry, may enable a diagnosis of non-GERD causes of esophageal symptoms in PPI-refractory patients (ie, achalasia or rumination). It is important to keep in mind the possibility of non-GERD causes (eg, achalasia, eosinophilic esophagitis [EoE], or a functional disorder) in PPI-refractory patients. In this context, endoscopy and reflux monitoring can be valuable tools to exclude GERD. The pros and cons of diagnostic modalities for GERD are summarized in **Table 1**. This article focuses primarily on patients with typical symptoms (heartburn or regurgitation) and discusses different modalities for the work up of GERD. A section summarizing the diagnostic approach for PPI-refractory symptoms, a common clinical problem, is also included.

DIAGNOSING GERD BY SYMPTOMS AND RESPONSE TO ACID SUPPRESSION

Heartburn and regurgitation are considered the most reliable symptoms for making a history-based diagnosis of GERD but are far from perfect in this respect.[3] In fact, these symptoms actually have variable sensitivity and specificity for diagnosing GERD.[4] Although heartburn is the most typical symptom of GERD, patients with heartburn represent a heterogeneous group; even if many or most of them have GERD, others may experience heartburn as a result of other esophageal disorders such as EoE or achalasia. Furthermore, some patients may have no organic cause for this symptom and are thus diagnosed with functional heartburn, one of the recognized functional gastrointestinal disorders.[5] GERD patients may also present with dysphagia, one of the alarm symptoms that warrants endoscopic evaluation to exclude a complication including malignancy. However, other potential causes for dysphagia must not be ignored. Chest pain may also be reported by GERD patients but this symptom requires thorough evaluation for cardiac disease before GERD is considered.

Recently, the spectrum of clinical presentations attributed to GERD has expanded beyond the typical esophageal symptoms of heartburn and regurgitation and now includes various extraesophageal manifestations, including asthma, chronic cough, and laryngitis.[6,7] However, a causal relationship between reflux and these extraesophageal presentations has been difficult to prove and these atypical symptoms frequently

Table 1
Pros and cons of diagnostic modalities for gastroesophageal reflux disease

Diagnostic Modality	Pros	Cons
PPI test	• Widely available • Simple • Noninvasive • Inexpensive	• Administration of test not standardized (PPI dose and duration vary) • Definition of response (partial vs complete) not standardized • Limited sensitivity and specificity
Endoscopy	• GERD can be diagnosed confidently when erosive esophagitis is present • Can diagnose non-GERD disorders such as EoE	• Invasive, often requiring sedation • A normal endoscopy (found in 2/3 of GERD patients) does not rule out GERD • Esophageal biopsies obtained during endoscopy are not useful to diagnose GERD
Reflux monitoring		
Catheter-based pH	• The gold standard for GERD diagnosis by assessing esophageal acid exposure • Positive test predicts response to therapy	• Catheter discomfort may limit diet and activities • Study restricted to 24 h • Unable to detect nonacid reflux (with pH>4)
Wireless pH	• Like catheter-pH, measures esophageal acid exposure • Better tolerability • Prolonged monitoring (up to 96 h)	• More costly than catheter-based techniques • Requires endoscopy for placement • Unable to detect nonacid reflux (with pH>4)
Impedance-pH	• Measures esophageal acid exposure • Can detect nonacid reflux	• Catheter discomfort may limit activities • Study restricted to 24 h • Analysis of tracings more laborious than pH alone

have multifactorial causes in which gastroesophageal reflux may be a cofactor instead of a cause. Extraesophageal syndromes rarely occur in isolation without concomitant typical symptoms of GERD.[8]

A variety of validated questionnaires have been developed for GERD, including specific symptom scales, quality of life scales, and those which combine the two. A comprehensive discussion of these instruments is outside the scope of this article. Although these instruments may be helpful, they have similar specificity and sensitivity to a clinical examination by a gastroenterologist and are usually reserved for screening large numbers of patients by personnel who are not specialists or as part of clinical trials.[9]

Although the limitations of heartburn and regurgitation for making a diagnosis of GERD should be recognized, it is not necessary to conduct a diagnostic evaluation in all patients with typical symptoms and no alarm features. For these patients, a short trial of acid suppression with a PPI represents a noninvasive, simple, and reasonable option for supporting a diagnosis of GERD. If the patient has a clear response to therapy, it can be assumed that GERD is present. That is not to say that the PPI test is without shortcomings. The manner in which this test is administered is not standardized, with differing PPI doses (once vs twice daily), variable duration of treatment (from 1 to 4 weeks), and different definitions of a positive response to PPI (either partial or complete). Moreover, a meta-analysis of several studies that evaluated the diagnostic capability of a short course of PPI compared with other diagnostic interventions, found a sensitivity of 78% and specificity of 54% for the PPI test.[10]

ESOPHAGRAM AND ESOPHAGEAL MANOMETRY

A diagnosis of GERD cannot be made based on the results of an esophagram or esophageal manometry. However, it is important to briefly discuss these tests because they are often used in the work-up of patients with symptoms suggestive of GERD.

The presence of erosive esophagitis may be documented through a high-quality barium esophagram but the overall sensitivity of this test for esophagitis is low.[11] The finding of reflux of barium from stomach to esophagus is frequently included in esophagram reports, with or without provocative maneuvers. However, this finding may be absent in GERD patients and it can be elicited with provocative maneuvers in some healthy patients.[12,13] An esophagram can be helpful when a patient has dysphagia because it may reveal a structural abnormality such as a stricture or ring; however, endoscopy has a higher yield for this purpose. In summary, a diagnosis of GERD cannot be made through esophagram.

GERD patients may show evidence of impaired peristalsis or a hypotensive lower esophageal sphincter during esophageal manometry[14] but these findings are not specific and may be found in the absence of GERD. In patients with esophageal symptoms (heartburn, regurgitation, chest pain, and dysphagia) attributed to GERD who do not respond to PPI therapy, manometry should be performed to rule out achalasia or other motor disorders.[3] Before antireflux surgery, esophageal manometry is mandatory to rule out achalasia or scleroderma-like esophagus because these conditions represent contraindications to fundoplication. The presence of decreased peristalsis before surgery is less important because this has not been found to reliably predict dysphagia following fundoplication.[15]

ENDOSCOPIC EVALUATION AND ROLE OF ESOPHAGEAL BIOPSIES

Upper endoscopy enables direct visualization of the esophageal mucosa and may reveal erosive esophagitis as well as stricture and Barrett esophagus. The most widely used system for grading the severity of esophagitis is the Los Angeles classification, which has been well validated in terms of interobserver variability.[16] GERD can be diagnosed with confidence when erosive esophagitis is found; however, endoscopy is normal in approximately two-thirds of patients with heartburn and regurgitation, and the absence of esophagitis does not rule out GERD.[17] Obtaining random esophageal biopsies as a means of diagnosing GERD in patients with normal endoscopy is not recommended because the so-called classic histologic findings of GERD (basal cell hyperplasia, papillary elongation, and infiltration with neutrophils or eosinophils) have poor diagnostic performance characteristics. These findings may be absent in disease, and present in non-GERD controls.[18,19] In the current era of increasing prevalence of EoE, random distal and proximal esophageal biopsies may be useful in patients without a clear diagnosis because EoE patients may present with symptoms that are similar to those experienced by GERD patients (heartburn, dysphagia, and chest pain). Importantly, endoscopy may appear normal (without the typical rings or linear furrows) in up to 10% of EoE patients.[20]

REFLUX MONITORING

Direct quantification of reflux is only possible by ambulatory, prolonged (at least 24 hours) reflux monitoring techniques, which represent the gold standard in the diagnosis of GERD. The main goal of a reflux monitoring test is to establish whether an abnormal, pathologic amount of reflux is present by measuring esophageal acid exposure or the number or reflux episodes. In addition, reflux monitoring offers an opportunity to assess the temporal relationship between reflux episodes and reported symptoms. Traditionally, reflux monitoring was performed through catheter-based pH measurements. Recent advances include the development of a wireless pH capsule that allows catheter-free monitoring and impedance-pH measurement, a catheter-based technique that enables detection of acid, as well as nonacid reflux (ie, with pH >4). Esophageal bilirubin monitoring has been used but is not routinely used in clinical practice and not widely available.[21] There are several catheters that incorporate pH monitoring at the level of the pharynx. However, pharyngeal pH monitoring has important shortcomings and it generally does not predict response to treatment.[22] A new transnasal pharyngeal catheter that is capable of detecting acid in liquid or aerosolized form has been developed[23] but data supporting its use are limited.

Catheter-Based and Wireless pH Monitoring

For many years the standard approach to ambulatory pH monitoring was to use a transnasal catheter to measure esophageal pH in the distal esophagus for 24 hours with a pH electrode positioned 5 cm above the proximal border of the lower esophageal sphincter. A reflux episode is defined by a drop in pH to below 4.0. A study of this nature enables several measurements, including the percentage of time during which esophageal pH is below 4 (acid exposure time), the number of reflux episodes, number of reflux episodes longer than 5 minutes, and longest reflux episode.[24] Of these, esophageal acid exposure is thought to be the most useful indicator of pathologic acid reflux.[25] A positive pH test can establish a diagnosis of GERD in a patient with normal endoscopy; it may also help to confirm or exclude GERD in patients who do not respond to PPI therapy. Although the sensitivity and specificity of this test are above 90% in some studies,[26,27] other data point to lower sensitivity.[28]

The presence of a transnasal catheter may result in changes in patient behavior such as altered eating habits and decreased activity.[29] To circumvent this issue and to allow for longer monitoring periods, a wireless pH monitoring capsule was developed. This capsule, which is attached to the distal esophagus during endoscopy, transmits pH data via radiofrequency signals to an external recording device worn on the patient's belt. Wireless pH monitoring has similar and possibly improved accuracy compared with catheter-based pH monitoring.[30] Not surprisingly, it is better tolerated than a transnasal catheter and results in less interference with diet and acitivity.[31,32] Furthermore, with the wireless pH capsule the standard is to perform monitoring for 48 hours and the test can be extended to up to 96 hours.[33] This prolonged monitoring period has been shown to improve sensitivity for distinguishing controls from subjects with GERD.[34]

Impedance-pH Monitoring

Both catheter-based and wireless capsule pH monitoring are focused on measuring acid reflux (ie, drops in pH to <4.0). However, these techniques do not allow assessment of nonacid reflux (ie, with pH >4), which may occur when the gastric contents are buffered (during pharmacologic acid suppression or in the postprandial period). Impedance-pH monitoring is the only available test that can measure acid as well as nonacid reflux. By measuring intraesophageal impedance in a series of conducting electrodes placed in a catheter that spans the length of the esophagus it is possible to detect movement of intraesophageal material in either antegrade or retrograde direction.[35] When coupled with a pH electrode (thus the term impedance-pH), these catheters enable very detailed characterization of gastroesophageal reflux episodes, including acidity (acid, nonacid), composition (air, liquid, or mixed), proximal extent (height), velocity, and clearance time. Impedance-pH is currently the most accurate and detailed method to measure gastroesophageal reflux.[36] During combined impedance and pH monitoring, impedance is used to detect retrograde bolus movement (ie, reflux), whereas pH measurement establishes the acidity of the reflux episode (acid if pH <4.0, nonacid otherwise). Nonacid reflux may be further classified as either weakly acidic (pH ≥4 but <7) or weakly alkaline (pH ≥7). During impedance-pH monitoring, reflux burden can be ascertained by measuring distal esophageal acid exposure or by the number of reflux episodes. Symptom association studies are performed by assessing the relationship between symptoms and all forms of reflux (acid and nonacid).

The main advantage of impedance-pH monitoring is the ability to detect nonacid reflux because acid reflux can be reliably measured by catheter-based or wireless pH monitoring. Therefore, the usefulness of impedance-pH monitoring is directly linked to the clinical relevance of nonacid reflux. It has been shown that nonacid reflux can cause symptoms that are indistinguishable from those caused by acid reflux.[37] As noted previously, nonacid reflux occurs only when the gastric contents are buffered, which is seen in the postprandial period or in patients who are receiving acid-suppressing medication. A recent systematic review found that in subjects on PPI therapy, most reflux episodes have a pH above 4. Furthermore, nonacid reflux is responsible for most reflux-related symptoms in subjects on PPI treatment.[38] Nonacid reflux can be treated by pharmacologic inhibition of transient lower esophageal sphincter relaxations[39] or through fundoplication.[40] However, there is a paucity of controlled studies examining the benefit of treating nonacid reflux. Therefore, although impedance-pH is considered the most accurate method for reflux detection, the clinical indications for its use and its role in managing GERD patients are still evolving while the merits of finding and treating nonacid reflux await confirmation by high-quality trials. Finally, even with available software, interpretation of impedance-pH tracings is usually more time consuming compared with pH monitoring tracings.

Beyond Reflux Burden: Symptom Association Studies During Reflux Monitoring

The main goal of reflux monitoring is to establish whether an abnormal amount of reflux is present. An additional goal may be to determine whether the patient's symptoms are indeed being caused by reflux episodes. The two most common methods to evaluate the temporal association between reflux episodes and symptoms are the symptom index (SI)[41] and the symptom association probability (SAP).[42] The SI is defined as the percentage of symptom events that are temporally related to a reflux episode (number of reflux-related symptom events/total number of symptom events × 100%). An SI of 50% is considered positive, meaning that the symptom is related to reflux. Although this value was derived from receiver operating characteristic (ROC) curves that found this threshold to be sensitive and specific for heartburn,[43] the SI is used to analyze any symptom that may be attributed to GERD. The SAP is calculated by dividing the pH or impedance-pH tracing in 2-minute segments and determining whether a reflux episode and/or a symptom occurred in each 2-minute segment. A 2 × 2 contingency table with the number of segments with and without symptoms and with and without reflux is built; the probability that a positive association between reflux and symptoms occurred by more than chance is evaluated through a modified chi-square test, with an SAP greater than 95% considered positive.

An in-depth discussion of the advantages and disadvantages of the SI and the SAP is beyond the scope of this article; however, it is important for clinicians to know that both have methodological shortcomings[44] and that symptom association studies are the least robust measure obtained during reflux monitoring. Regardless of whether SI or SAP is used, precise and timely symptom recording by the patient is needed along with accurate reflux detection by the testing device. Furthermore, prospective data to validate the ability of these symptom association measures to predict response to treatment are scarce. Nevertheless, during patient management, a strongly positive SI or SAP may suggest the need for a therapeutic intervention and a negative result supports the notion that the patient's symptoms are unlikely to be due to reflux. However, given the limitations of these measures, recent guidelines recommend that the SI and SAP should not be used in isolation and other reflux monitoring parameters, as well as the patient's overall presentation, should be taken into account.[3]

WORK UP OF PATIENTS WITH PPI-REFRACTORY SYMPTOMS

A frequent reason for consultation to gastroenterology is failure to achieve satisfactory symptom improvement after treatment with PPI. PPI-refractory patients are heterogeneous but may fall into one of four general categories: (1) true PPI failure with ongoing symptoms due to persistent reflux of acidic gastric material (acid reflux), (2) adequate acid gastric suppression by the PPI but frequent reflux of nonacidic material as the cause of the symptoms, (3) symptoms due to other disorders (eg, EoE or achalasia), (4) no organic cause for the symptoms (ie, a functional gastrointestinal disorder such as functional heartburn). Because, clearly, not all patients who fail to respond to PPIs have GERD, a very important goal of the diagnostic evaluation in these patients is to differentiate those with persistent reflux as the cause of the ongoing symptoms from those with non-GERD etiologies.

The first step in the management of PPI-refractory patients is to confirm compliance and ensure that dosing and timing of medication are adequate. Once compliance and appropriate dosing are ensured, a single trial of a different PPI can be considered. A randomized controlled trial in subjects with persistent GERD symptoms despite a single daily dose of PPI, showed that increasing PPI to twice daily or switching to another PPI resulted in symptomatic improvement in roughly 20% of subjects, without a clear advantage for either strategy.[45]

Patients with persistent symptoms despite optimization of PPI therapy require further work-up. Endoscopy is recommended for typical esophageal symptoms to look for erosive esophagitis (rare in acid-suppressed patients) and exclude nonreflux esophageal disorders such as EoE. If endoscopy is negative, as is frequently the case, reflux monitoring is indicated. Reflux monitoring should also be considered in patients with extraesophageal symptoms that persist despite PPI optimization and in whom non-GERD causes have been ruled out through pulmonary, ears-nose-throat, and allergy evaluation.

Two important issues to weigh when preparing to perform reflux monitoring are whether the test should be done while on PPI therapy or after cessation of this medication, and what tool to use (catheter-based pH, wireless pH, or impedance-pH). Reflux monitoring off PPI (7 days after stopping therapy) can be performed with any of the available techniques (catheter, wireless pH, or impedance-pH) because the main goal is to measure acid reflux. Reflux monitoring on PPI should be performed with impedance-pH monitoring to enable measurement of nonacid reflux. The yield of pH monitoring without impedance in a patient taking a PPI is very low because in acid-suppressed patients reflux becomes predominantly nonacid.[37]

Studies comparing the yield of off-therapy with on-therapy reflux monitoring in refractory GERD patients are limited and inconclusive. For instance, Hemmink and colleagues[46] concluded that testing should be performed off PPI; in contrast, Pritchett and colleagues[47] found that reflux monitoring on PPI may be the preferred strategy. Not surprisingly, there is no clear consensus regarding the optimal testing approach for patients with PPI-refractory symptoms. One option is to stop medication in all such patients so that GERD can be either confirmed or ruled out. Patients without GERD can go on to testing and treatment of other causes, including functional disorders, whereas those with confirmed GERD can undergo escalation of therapy and further diagnostic interventions, possibly including reflux monitoring while on PPI to assess for ongoing acid or nonacid reflux. A second option, suggested in recent guidelines,[3,25] is to base the approach to testing on the patient's clinical presentation and pretest likelihood of GERD (**Fig. 1**). Patients with low likelihood of GERD (eg, complete absence of response to PPI, extraesophageal presentations without concomitant typical symptoms) may be tested off therapy. If the test is negative, GERD is excluded and other causes are pursued. Patients with high likelihood of GERD (eg, at least partial response to PPI, typical symptoms, other features to suggest GERD such as large hiatus hernia) may be tested while on therapy in search of reflux (acid or nonacid) that persists despite acid suppression. In the latter patients, off-PPI reflux monitoring has reasonable likelihood to be positive but this finding will not provide information regarding the reason for the ongoing symptoms. In some patients, testing both off as well as on therapy is necessary to clarify the reason for PPI-refractoriness.

Finally, it is important to stress the importance of stopping PPI therapy in patients with refractory symptoms in whom all testing is negative. In a recent study, after a negative evaluation for refractory GERD that included normal endoscopy and impedance-pH monitoring, 42% of 90 subjects reported continued use of PPI despite negative results.[48] This study highlights the importance of educating the patient about the need to stop PPIs after the work-up is negative for GERD.

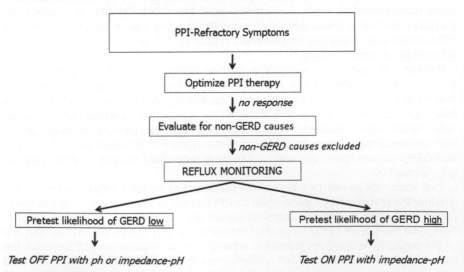

Fig. 1. Suggested work up for patients with PPI-refractory symptoms. (*Adapted from Katz PO, Gerson L, Vela MF. Guidelines for the diagnosis and management of gastroesophageal reflux disease. Am J Gastroenterol 2013;108:322; with permission.*)

SUMMARY

GERD may be diagnosed based on symptoms and a positive response to acid suppression (the PPI test) in patients with typical presentations and no alarm features. However, it is important to be aware of the limited sensitivity and specificity of this approach as a diagnostic intervention. Patients with alarm features such as dysphagia or weight loss and those with typical symptoms and incomplete response to PPI, should undergo endoscopy. When endoscopy reveals erosive esophagitis, GERD can be diagnosed confidently; however, most patients have normal endoscopic evaluation. Esophageal biopsies to diagnose GERD based on histologic findings are not recommended because of the poor diagnostic capability of these findings. Reflux monitoring can document the presence of pathologic reflux and may shed light on the relationship between reflux episodes and reported symptoms. Monitoring by pH relies on detecting acid reflux, either by catheter technique or with a wireless capsule. Impedance-pH monitoring is required when there is a need to measure nonacid reflux (ie, with a pH >4), which may be clinically important in patients who do not improve with PPI therapy. Patients with persistent symptoms despite PPI are a heterogeneous group. These patients may have ongoing reflux (acid or nonacid) as the cause of their symptoms, they may have non-GERD disorders such as EoE or achalasia, or they may have a functional gastrointestinal disorder. There is no consensus regarding whether testing of refractory patients should be performed on versus off therapy. One option is to use the pretest likelihood of GERD to guide testing: those with low likelihood of GERD should be tested off therapy, whereas those with high likelihood of GERD should be tested on PPI. For PPI-refractory patients in whom GERD is ruled out, PPI should be discontinued and other causes need to be investigated.

REFERENCES

1. Locke GR III, Talley NJ, Fett SL, et al. Prevalence and clinical spectrum of gastro-esophageal reflux: a population-based study in Olmsted County, Minnesota. Gastroenterology 1997;112:1448–56.
2. Lind T, Havelund T, Carlsson R, et al. Heartburn without esophagitis: efficacy of omeprazole therapy and features determining therapeutic response. Scand J Gastroenterol 1997;32:974–9.
3. Katz PO, Gerson L, Vela MF. Guidelines for the diagnosis and management of gastroesophageal reflux disease. Am J Gastroenterol 2013;108:308–28.
4. Klauser AG, Shcindelbeck NE, Muller-Lissner SA. Symptoms in gastro-oesophageal reflux disease. Lancet 1990;335:205.
5. Zerbib F, Bruley de Varannes S, Simon M, et al. Functional heartburn: definition and management strategies. Curr Gastroenterol Rep 2012;14:181–8.
6. Irwin RS, Curley FJ, French CL. Chronic cough. The spectrum and frequency of causes, key components of the diagnostic evaluation, and outcome of specific therapy. Am Rev Respir Dis 1990;141:640–7.
7. El-Serag HB, Sonnenberg A. Comorbid occurrence of laryngeal or pulmonary disease with esophagitis in United States military veterans. Gastroenterology 1997;113:755–60.
8. Vakil N, van Zanten SV, Kahrilas P, et al. The Montreal definition and classification of gastroesophageal reflux disease: a global evidence-based consensus. Am J Gastroenterol 2006;101:1900.
9. Stanghellini V, Arsmtrong D, Monnikes H, et al. Systematic review; do we need a new gastroesophageal diseases questionnaire. Digestion 2007;75(suppl 1):3–16.

10. Numans ME, Lau J, de Wit NK, et al. Short-term treatment with proton-pump inhibitors as a test for gastroesophageal reflux disease. Ann Intern Med 2004;140: 518–52.
11. Johnston BT, Troshinsky MB, Castell JA, et al. Comparison of barium radiology with esophageal pH monitoring in the diagnosis of gastroesophageal reflux disease. Am J Gastroenterol 1996;91:1181–5.
12. Thompson JK, Koehler RE, Richter JE. Detection of gastroesophageal reflux: value of barium studies compared with 24-hr pH monitoring. Am J Roentgenol 1994;162:621–6.
13. Richter JE, Castell DO. Gastroesophageal reflux. Pathogenesis, diagnosis, and therapy. Ann Intern Med 1982;97:93–103.
14. Savarino E, Gemignani L, Pohl D, et al. Oesophageal motility and bolus transit abnormalities increase in parallel with the severity of gastro-oesophageal reflux disease. Aliment Pharmacol Ther 2011;34:476–86.
15. Shaw JM, Bornman PC, Callanan MD, et al. Long-term outcome of laparoscopic Nissen and laparoscopic Toupet fundoplication for gastroesophageal reflux disease: a prospective, randomized trial. Surg Endosc 2010;24:924–32.
16. Lundell LR, Dent J, Bennett JR, et al. Endoscopic assessment of oesophagitis: clinical and functional correlates and further validation of the Los Angeles classification. Gut 1999;45:172–80.
17. Johnsson F, Joelsson B, Gudmundsson K, et al. Symptoms and endoscopic findings in the diagnosis of gastroesophageal reflux disease. Scand J Gastroenterol 1987;22:714–8.
18. Nandurkar S, Talley NJ, Martin CJ, et al. Esophageal histology does not provide additional useful information over clinical assessment in identifying reflux patients presenting for esophagogastroduodenoscopy. Dig Dis Sci 2000;2000(45): 217–24.
19. Tytgat G. The value of esophageal histology in the diagnosis of gastroesophageal reflux disease in patients with heartburn and normal endoscopy. Curr Gastroenterol Rep 2008;10:231–4.
20. Prasad GA, Talley NJ, Romero Y, et al. Prevalence and predictive factors of eosinophilic esophagitis in patients presenting with dysphagia: a prospective study. Am J Gastroenterol 2007;102:2627.
21. Vaezi MF, Richter JE. Role of acid and duodenogastroesophageal reflux in gastroesophageal reflux disease. Gastroenterology 1996;111:1192–9.
22. Vaezi MF, Hicks DM, Abelson TI, et al. Laryngeal signs and symptoms of gastroesophageal reflux disease (GERD): a critical assessment of cause and effect association. Clin Gastroenterol Hepatol 2003;1:333–44.
23. Sun G, Muddana S, Slaughter JC, et al. A new pH catheter for laryngopharyngeal reflux: Normal values. Laryngoscope 2009;119:1639–43.
24. Johnson LF, Demeester TR. Twenty-four-hour pH monitoring of the distal esophagus. A quantitative measure of gastroesophageal reflux. Am J Gastroenterol 1974;62:325–32.
25. Pandolfino JE, Vela MF. Esophageal reflux monitoring. Gastrointest Endosc 2009; 69:917–30.
26. Jamieson JR, Stein HJ, DeMeester TR, et al. Ambulatory 24-h esophageal pH monitoring: normal values, optimal thresholds, specificity, sensitivity, and reproducibility. Am J Gastroenterol 1992;87:1102–11.
27. Richter JE, Bradley LA, DeMeester TR, et al. Normal 24-hr ambulatory esophageal pH values. Influence of study center, pH electrode, age, and gender. Dig Dis Sci 1992;37:849–56.

28. Schlesinger PK, Donahue PE, Schmid B, et al. Limitations of 24-hour intraesophageal pH monitoring in the hospital setting. Gastroenterology 1985;894:797–804.
29. Fass R, Hell R, Sampliner RE, et al. Effect of ambulatory 24-h esophageal pH monitoring on reflux-provoking activities. Dig Dis Sci 1999;44:2263–9.
30. Pandolfino J, Zhang Q, Schreiner M, et al. Acid reflux event detection using the Bravo™ wireless vs the Slimline™ catheter pH systems: why are the numbers so different? Gut 2005;54:1687–92.
31. Wenner J, Jonsson F, Johansson J, et al. Wireless esophageal pH monitoring is better tolerated than the catheter-based technique: results from a randomized cross-over trial. Am J Gastroenterol 2007;102:239–45.
32. Ward EM, Devault KR, Bouras EP, et al. Successful oesophageal pH monitoring with a catheter-free system. Aliment Pharmacol Ther 2004;19:449–54.
33. Hirano I, Zhang Q, Pandolfino JE, et al. Four-day Bravo pH capsule monitoring with and without proton pump inhibitor therapy. Clin Gastroenterol Hepatol 2005;3:1083–8.
34. Pandolfino JE, Richter JE, Ours T, et al. Ambulatory esophageal pH monitoring using a wireless system. Am J Gastroenterol 2003;984:740–9.
35. Vela MF. Non-acid reflux: detection by multichannel intraluminal impedance and pH, clinical significance and management. Am J Gastroenterol 2009;104:277–80.
36. Sifrim D, Castell D, Dent J, et al. Gastro-oesophageal reflux monitoring: reflux and consensus report on detection and definitions of acid, non-acid, and gas reflux. Gut 2004;53:1024–31.
37. Vela MF, Camacho-Lobato L, Srinivasan R, et al. Intraesophageal impedance and pH measurement of acid and non-acid reflux: effect of omeprazole. Gastroenterology 2001;96:647–55.
38. Boeckxstaens GE, Smout A. Systematic review: role of acid, weakly acidic and weakly alkaline reflux in gastro-oesophageal reflux disease. Aliment Pharmacol ther 2010;32:334–43.
39. Vela MF, Tutuian R, Katz PO, et al. Baclofen decreases acid and non-acid postprandial gastro-oesophageal reflux measured by combined multichannel intraluminal impedance and pH. Aliment Pharmacol Ther 2003;17:243–51.
40. Frazzoni M, Conigliaro R, Melotti G. Reflux parameters as modified by laparoscopic fundoplication in 40 patients with heartburn/regurgitation persisting despite PPI therapy: a study using impedance-pH monitoring. Dig Dis Sci 2011;56:1099–106.
41. Wiener GJ, Richter JE, Copper JB, et al. The symptom index: a clinically important parameter of ambulatory 24-hour esophageal pH monitoring. Am J Gastroenterol 1988;83:358–61.
42. Weusten BL, Roelofs JM, Akkermans LM, et al. The symptom-association probability: an improved method for symptom analysis of 24-hour esophageal pH data. Gastroenterology 1994;107:1741–5.
43. Singh S, Richter JE, Bradley LA, et al. The symptom index. Differential usefulness in suspected acid-related complaints of heartburn and chest pain. Dig Dis Sci 1993;34:309–16.
44. Connor J, Richter J. Increasing yield also increases false positives and best serves to exclude GERD. Am J Gastroenterol 2006;101:460–3.
45. Fass R, Murthy U, Hayden CW, et al. Omeprazole 40 mg once a day is equally effective as lansoprazole 30 mg twice a day in symptom control of patients with gastro-oesophageal reflux disease (GERD) who are resistant to conventional-dose lansoprazole therapy-a prospective, randomized, multi-centre study. Aliment Pharmacol Ther 2000;14:1595–603.

46. Hemmink GJ, Bredenoord AJ, Weusten BL, et al. Esophageal pH-impedance monitoring in patients with therapy-resistant reflux symptoms: 'on' or 'off' proton pump inhibitor? Am J Gastroenterol 2008;103:2446–53.
47. Pritchett JM, Aslam M, Slaughter JC, et al. Efficacy of esophageal impedance/pH monitoring in patients with refractory gastroesophageal reflux disease, on and off therapy. Clin Gastroenterol Hepatol 2009;7:743–8.
48. Gawron AJ, Rothe J, Fought AJ, et al. Many patients continue using proton pump inhibitors after negative results from tests for reflux disease. Clin Gastroenterol Hepatol 2012;10:620–5.

Esophageal Function Testing

Beyond Manometry and Impedance

Ravinder K. Mittal, MD

KEYWORDS

- Manometry • Achalasia • Impedence • Esophagus
- Longitudinal muscle esophagus • US imaging esophagus

KEY POINTS

- Manometry and impedance provide information regarding circular muscle function and luminal content respectively.
- Ultrasound imaging provides a unique perspective of esophageal function by providing important information regarding longitudinal muscle contraction, coordination between the two muscle layers of muscularis propria and esophageal distension during bolus transport.
- Laser Doppler assessment of perfusion may be an important complementary tool to assess blood perfusion of esophageal wall as a possible mechanism of pain.

INTRODUCTION

Endoscopy, barium swallow, high-resolution manometry (HRM), pH measurement (either catheter based or using Bravo system), and impedance monitoring of the esophagus are major esophageal function testing techniques that are available in most academic centers and centers of excellence for esophageal function testing. These recording techniques provide key information on the sensory and motor functions of the esophagus that allows one to treat patients based on the physiologic understanding of the patient's symptoms. Another esophageal function testing technique, which even though has not gained wide popularity and acceptance, is ultrasound (US) imaging of the esophagus using either catheter-based intravascular US imaging probe or US endoscope. The latter is suited for anatomic/morphologic information of the esophageal muscle and identification of lesions that affect esophageal

Financial Support: This work was supported by National Institutes of Health Grant R01DK060733.

Conflict of Interest: Author has no conflict of interest.

Division of Gastroenterology, Department of Medicine, San Diego VA Health Care System, University of California, Gastroenterology (111D), 3350, La Jolla Village Drive, San Diego, CA 92161, USA

E-mail address: rmittal@ucsd.edu

function by compression of the esophagus. On the other hand, catheter-based US imaging provides information on anatomy/morphology as well as functional aspects of esophageal muscle function. In order for US imaging, especially dynamic US imaging, to gain popularity it will have to be user friendly and less expensive. To date, dynamic US imaging has only been used in research laboratories. There is no question though that the static and dynamic US imaging, using either US endoscopes or catheter-based US probes, provides key information of esophageal functions that is unparallel to any other technique.

Laser Doppler blood perfusion measurement of the esophageal wall is another important modality, especially if future testing confirms that "noncardiac" chest pain and proton pump inhibition (PPI)-resistant heartburn are related to low blood perfusion or relative ischemia of the esophageal wall. The goal of this writing is to provide principles underlying these techniques and to update the status of information that these techniques have yielded.

ULTRASOUND IMAGING OF ESOPHAGUS

The esophagus is no exception—like the rest of the gastrointestinal tract, its outer muscular coat or muscularis propria is organized into an outer longitudinal and an inner circular muscle layer. Recent studies prove that the longitudinal muscles of the esophagus play an important role in the physiology and pathophysiology of the sensory and motor function of the esophagus and one can study longitudinal muscle function using dynamic US imaging. The esophageal longitudinal muscle starts proximally as 3 bundles: (1) a main longitudinal muscle bundle that originates from the posterior surface of the cricoid cartilage, (2) an accessory muscle bundle from the posterolateral surface of cricoid cartilage, and (3) an accessory muscle bundle from the contralateral surface of the cricopharyngeus muscle. Muscle bundles from the 2 sides quickly fan out to surround the entire circumference of the esophagus, leaving only a triangular space, the area of Laimer that is not surrounded by the longitudinal muscle at the most cranial end of the esophagus. At the caudal end, longitudinal muscle fibers continue into the stomach and some may be inserted in the circular muscle bundles of the lower esophageal sphincter (LES). Contraction of the longitudinal muscles causes axial shortening of esophagus. Circular muscles of the esophagus do not travel in a perfectly circular fashion along the length of the esophagus, instead they are oriented in the helical fashion, especially in the distal part of the esophagus.[1–3] The angle of these helices increases as one goes toward the distal direction. Because of the helical morphology of circular muscle,[3] part of the axial esophageal shortening during peristalsis is the result of circular muscle contraction. Unlike circular muscle contraction and relaxations, which can be easily recorded by intraluminal pressure probes/manometry, it is difficult to measure contraction and relaxation of the longitudinal muscle. Dynamic US imaging provides information on the local longitudinal muscle contraction and axial shortening of the esophagus.[4]

In the animal experiments, longitudinal muscle contraction can be recorded by surgically implanted strain gauges in the long axis of the esophagus.[5] Longitudinal muscle contraction can also be recorded by radio-opaque markers implanted in the long axis of esophagus (in humans[6,7] and animals[8]) in combination with radiographic fluoroscopy, which records motion of the radio-opaque markers as a proxy of longitudinal muscle contraction. Clearly, these studies have provided important information; however they are of limited use for the human experimentation for several obvious reasons: (1) strain gauze implantation is not practical and (2) radiation exposure for prolonged recordings limits use of radio-opaque marker technique. More recently, a sensor that uses magnet and electromagnetic field (Hall effect) has been used to study axial motions of the squamocolumnar junction/esophagogastric junction, as an indirect marker of longitudinal muscle contraction of the esophagus.[9] One of the limitations of all of the methods mentioned earlier is that they do not record longitudinal muscle contraction at one site (local contraction) in the esophagus, like manometry does for circular muscle.

US imaging performed using thin (1–2 mm diameter) intravascular catheters can record longitudinal muscle contraction at a focal point in the esophagus over extended time periods.[10,11] US imaging also provides other important information, that is, esophageal muscle hypertrophy and luminal distension during peristalsis and gastroesophageal reflux (GER), key esophageal functions that cannot be measured by other modalities. For recording longitudinal muscle contraction, US imaging relies on the "law of mass conservation", that is, when esophagus shortens in length (axial shortening) it causes a proportional increase in the esophageal muscle cross-sectional area and muscle thickness, which can be visualized and quantitated by US image analysis. The strength of US imaging techniques is that the recording can be done in humans for extended time periods. The major limitations of US imaging are that the equipment is expensive and data analysis is time consuming. The methodology to record US imaging and data analysis has been described in detail in an earlier publication.[11]

STATIC US IMAGING
Muscle Hypertrophy in Esophageal Motor Disorders and Its Significance

US imaging, endoscope-based or catheter-based, provides important information of the esophageal muscle thickness in the resting or baseline condition. In normal subjects, both circular and longitudinal muscles are relatively thin (0.75 mm each).[10,12] Muscle thickness is greater in the distal esophagus and it decreases in the proximal direction.[13] Atropine decreases baseline muscle thickness,[14] which suggests presence of baseline tone in the circular and longitudinal muscles of the esophagus and confirm early studies that used esophageal barostat to measure esophageal tone. Using echo endoscopes, several investigators reported case reports of marked muscle hypertrophy in patients with nonspecific motor disorders and nutcracker esophagus. Systematic assessment of patients with various types of esophageal motor disorders revealed interesting differences in muscle thickness between normal subjects and patients, as well as among patients with various types of motility disorders. Patients with primary or idiopathic motor disorders in general have an increase in the thickness of both circular and longitudinal muscle layers, even though the circular muscle thickness is greater than the longitudinal muscle.[11] The increase in muscle thickness is seen primarily in the distal esophagus and it decreases gradually from distal to the proximal end. Another important finding is that the degree of muscle thickness increase or in other words muscle hypertrophy differs in different motor disorders; generally it follows (not always) the following pattern: muscle thickness in achalasia esophagus > diffuse esophageal spasm > nutcracker esophagus > nonspecific motor disorders (**Fig. 1**). In the case of a distended esophagus, like in achalasia esophagus, muscle thickness decreases as esophagus becomes dilated; however, the cross-sectional area of muscle that represents the muscle mass is significantly larger in achalasia esophagus than other motor disorders. In a study of 98 consecutive patients referred to the motility laboratory for various symptoms, simultaneous manometry and US imaging were performed to determine the relationship between various motility disorders and muscle hypertrophy.[15] Nearly all patients with primary motility disorders, based

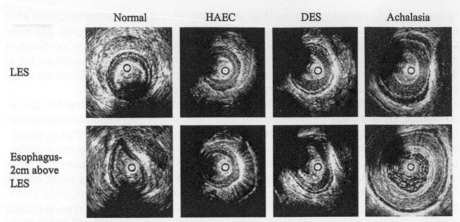

Fig. 1. Muscle hypertrophy in esophageal motor disorders: US images of the LES and esophageal body in healthy subjects and patients with high-amplitude esophageal contractions (HAEC), diffuse esophageal spasm (DES), and achalasia of the esophagus. The LES image is from the center of the LES. The esophageal images are from a time when there was no esophageal contractile activity, which was observed through manometry. Note the differences in the muscle thickness in 4 subjects, with the thickest muscle in patients with achalasia of the esophagus. (*From* Dogan I, Puckett JL, Padda BS, et al. Prevalence of increased esophageal muscle thickness in patients with esophageal symptoms. Am J Gastroenterol 2007;102:137–45; with permission.)

on manometry, were found to have an increased thickness of muscularis propria. Interestingly, 25% of patients with normal esophageal manometry also had thicker esophageal muscle than normal subject, albeit of smaller magnitude than seen in patients with typical motility disorders. Even though manometry has been normal in these patients, they had esophageal symptoms of dysphagia, chest pain, and heartburn. One interpretation of these findings is that normal manometry does not guarantee normal esophageal function, and US imaging could be a more sensitive technique than manometry to detect esophageal motor dysfunction.

What does an increase in muscle thickness signify and what is its relevance? Major cause of increase in muscle thickness/muscle hypertrophy in all muscles is overactivity or contraction of the muscle against resistance (afterload). For example, systemic hypertension and aortic stenosis cause hypertrophy of the left ventricle. Animal studies show that outflow obstruction to the esophagus induces hypertrophy/increase in esophageal muscle thickness and alteration in esophageal motor function that is not dissimilar to the one seen in association with primary/idiopathic spastic motor disorders. It may be that the fundamental abnormality in primary/idiopathic motor disorders lies in the LES function, which does not either relax or open up normally, and changes in the esophageal motor function are secondary to the LES dysfunction. The degree of LES dysfunction may determine the severity of esophageal motor dysfunction and muscle hypertrophy. For example, the LES dysfunction is most severe in achalasia esophagus and so is the esophageal body dysfunction and so on. Another pathologic process that causes muscle hypertrophy is inflammation, for example, patients with Crohn disease have hypertrophy of muscles of small intestine. Transforming growth factor-β1 and related growth factors are key players in the inflammation-induced muscle hypertrophy.[16] It is unlikely though that inflammation plays an important role in esophageal muscle hypertrophy because types of inflammation that afflicts the esophagus, that is, reflux-induced esophagitis and eosinophilic esophagitis are not associated with an increase in the muscle thickness. To the contrary, muscle thickness is reduced in patients with reflux esophagitis and it is not altered significantly in eosinophilic esophagitis.[17] Systemic sclerosis or scleroderma esophagus is associated with loss of muscle mass and decrease in the esophageal muscle thickness.[18]

DYNAMIC US IMAGING
Patterns of Longitudinal Muscle Contraction in Health and Their Significance to Normal Esophageal Function

Dynamic US imaging of the esophagus is performed using catheter-based, intravascular US probes that are 1 to 2 mm in diameter. They were designed initially to study coronary arteries. These catheters can be easily placed via nose into the esophagus. Using these probes, US imaging of the esophagus can be performed continuously for hours; we have recorded US images for up to 24 hours.[19] Images are usually recorded on a videotape, digitized, and then analyzed, even though one can record images in the digital format directly without using videotape. US images recorded by current systems are cross-sectional/tomographic/B-mode images that can be converted into M-mode US images to display changes in muscle thickness over time.[20] These M-mode US images then can be superimposed on the manometry or other types of recordings to determine the relationship between changes in pressure or other parameters of interest and changes in the muscle thickness. Manometry studies show that during esophageal peristalsis, certain length or a segment of the esophagus, rather than a point location, contracts in a peristaltic or sequential fashion. This segment of circular muscle contraction progresses sequentially from oral to aboral direction. The length of the contracted segment increases as it moves in the caudal direction.[21] Pressure in the contracted segment is distributed in the form of a bell-shaped curve with peak pressure in its middle. US images show that the longitudinal muscle contracts in harmony with the circular muscle; the 2 are precisely coordinated in location and timing.[20] The peak of contraction in the circular and longitudinal layer occurs within 1 second of each other (**Figs. 2** and **3**). Distension of a balloon in the esophagus also induces contraction and relaxation of the 2 muscle layers, cranial and caudal to the site of distension, respectively.[22] However, that does not mean that the 2 layers cannot contract independent of each other; for example, during transient LES relaxation, a key motor event that allows retrograde transport of gastric contents into the esophagus (vomiting, belching, and reflux) pattern of contraction in the 2 muscle layers is different from peristalsis.[23,24] Just before the onset of transient LES relaxation, longitudinal muscle contracts independent of circular muscle, starting at the caudal end of the esophagus and it marches in the oral direction. Longitudinal muscle contraction during transient LES relaxation is significantly greater in amplitude and longer in duration than during peristalsis. Another distinct pattern of longitudinal muscle contraction is seen in association with subthreshold stimulation of pharynx during which there is also relaxation of the LES.[25] Longitudinal muscle contracts only at the cranial end of the esophagus, that is, just caudal to the upper esophageal sphincter with subthreshold pharyngeal stimulus. These findings prove that the 2 layers can contract together during peristalsis and independent of each other during transient LES relaxation. Recent studies also prove that the 2 muscle layers are not anchored/cemented to each other, rather they slide against each other during peristalsis and transient LES relaxation (Patel N, Bhargava V, Kim HS, et al. Differential axial shortening of circular and longitudinal muscle during peristalsis and transient lower esophageal sphincter relaxation. Submitted for publication.). Interestingly, they slide in the

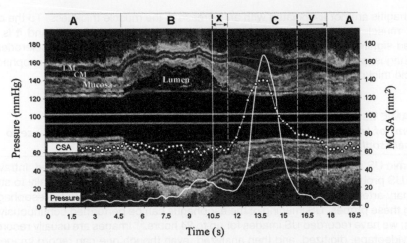

Fig. 2. Coordination of esophageal circular and longitudinal muscles during peristalsis: M-mode echo-esophagraph with superimposed, intraesophageal pressure and muscle cross-sectional area (MCSA) during 5-mL water swallow; US transducer positioned 2 cm above the lower esophageal sphincter. (A) Baseline esophagus, before swallow; (B) bolus-induced distension bolus pressure, thinning of mucosa and muscle layers; (C) esophageal contraction. Note the dissociation between increase in MCSA and increase in intraluminal pressure. The increase in MCSA (—o—) begins before and outlasts the intraluminal pressure wave (——). The difference between the onset of CSA and pressure is due to the delay in recording circular muscle contraction by manometry. CM, circular muscle; LM, longitudinal muscle. (*From* Mittal RK, Padda B, Bhalla V, et al. Synchrony between circular and longitudinal muscle contractions during peristalsis in normal subjects. Am J Physiol Gastrointest Liver Physiol 2006;290:G431–8; with permission.)

opposite direction during these 2 motor events, that is, there is greater axial shortening of the circular muscle than the longitudinal muscle during peristalsis and reverse is the case during transient LES relaxation.

Occlusion of the lumen caused by circular muscle contraction and its sequential aboral or oral progression (peristalsis or reverse peristalsis) causes bolus propulsion and retropulsion, respectively. Then what does longitudinal muscle layer, which comprises 50% of the muscle mass of the muscularis propria do? Longitudinal muscle contraction and relaxation results in thickening and thinning of the 2 muscle layers respectively,[11,22] which provide distinct mechanical advantages. Increase in muscle thickness reduces esophageal wall stress[26] and compliance in the contracted segment, both of which are important for esophageal lumen occlusion, which is an essential element for the bolus propulsion. On the other hand, decrease in esophageal wall thickness in the relaxed segment increases esophageal wall compliance that is also an essential requirement for the bolus propulsion. Another important function of longitudinal muscle contraction is that it causes lengthening of the esophageal segment distal to the site of contraction[6] and axial pull on the LES in the oral direction. Recent studies prove that a pull of the LES in the oral direction induces neurally mediated relaxation of the LES.[27,28] Along the same lines, it is likely that elongation of esophageal segment distal to contraction site induces its active relaxation (descending relaxation).[29] Relaxation of esophagus and LES distal to the site of contraction allows contracted segment to propel bolus with minimal resistance (see **Fig. 3**). Relaxation of the esophagus distal to the site of the contraction and resulting increase in esophageal wall compliance allow distension of the

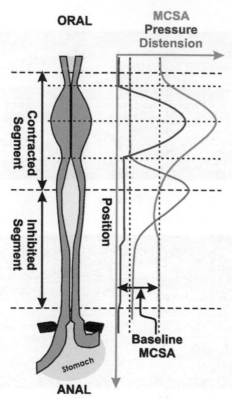

Fig. 3. Schematic of contraction and distension during swallow-induced peristalsis: note that the pressure and MCSA, surrogate markers of circular and longitudinal muscle contractions, respectively, precede distension. The latter marches distally in front of the onset of contraction wave in a peristaltic fashion. (*From* Abrahao L Jr, Bhargava V, Babaei A, et al. Swallow induces a peristaltic wave of distension that marches in front of the peristaltic wave of contraction. Neurogastroenterol Motil 2011;23:201–7, e110; with permission.)

esophagus. The degree of distension of the esophagus during peristalsis is an indirect marker of active relaxation of esophagus. US imaging allows quantitation of luminal distension. Studies show that similar to contraction, active relaxation of esophagus also occurs in a peristaltic fashion thus allowing bolus to move efficiently during peristalsis.

PATTERNS OF LONGITUDINAL MUSCLE CONTRACTION IN THE DISEASED STATES

As pointed earlier, during normal peristalsis longitudinal and circular muscles contract in a synchronous fashion, with peak contraction of the 2 muscle layers occurring within 1 second of each other. An increase in cholinergic activity, that is, administration of acetylcholinesterase inhibitor (edrophonium), induces disassociation between the 2 muscle layers so that the peak longitudinal muscle contraction occurs before the peak circular muscle contraction.[30] In patients with nutcracker esophagus, which appears to be a hypercholinergic state, there is spontaneous disassociation between contractions of the 2 muscle layers. Peak contraction of the 2 muscle layers is separated by several seconds[31] in nutcracker esophagus (**Fig. 4**). Interestingly, the disassociation between the 2 muscle layers is abolished by atropine (an anticholinergic

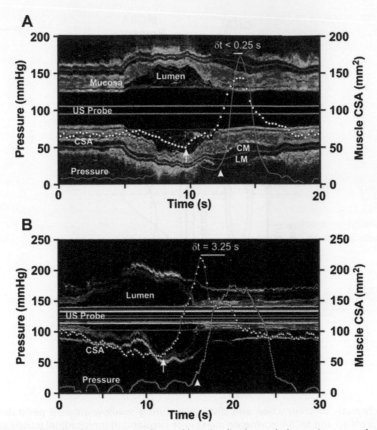

Fig. 4. Discoordination between circular and longitudinal muscle layers in nutcracker esophagus. (*A*) Relationship between M-mode US images, MCSA, and the pressure wave in a normal subject. Note that the onset of lumen collapse occurs at the same time as the onset of the increase in MCSA (*arrow*). Pressure wave (*arrowhead*) occurs at the same time as the first complete collapse of the lumen on the manometric probe. Peak of manometric contraction and peak CSA occurred with a delta-t less than or equal to 0.5 s during all 28 swallows at the 2 cm and all 28 swallows at the 10-cm level. (*B*) An example of dissociation between CM and LM muscle contraction in a patient with nutcracker esophagus. These recordings were obtained at 2 cm above the lower esophageal sphincter. Note the disassociation between the peak pressure and peak MCSA. (*From* Jung HY, Puckett JL, Bhalla V, et al. Asynchrony between the circular and the longitudinal muscle contraction in patients with nutcracker esophagus. Gastroenterology 2005;128:1179–86; with permission.)

agent) in patients with nutcracker esophagus[32]; which suggests that nutcracker esophagus represents a hypercholinergic state that on one hand induces high amplitude contraction and on the other it causes a disassociation between the 2 muscles layers. An immunohistochemistry study found an increase in the expression of muscarinic receptors on the esophageal muscles in patients with nutcracker esophagus.[33] How does discoordination in the 2 layers cause esophageal symptoms? Although this is not entirely clear, it may be that discoordination between the 2 layers interferes with descending relaxation or distension of esophagus, thus causing relative narrowing of esophagus, which impedes with the bolus propulsion. Dysphagia, an important symptom in patients with nutcracker esophagus, may be related to discoordination between the 2 layers.

Another example of the discoordination between longitudinal and circular muscle layers is seen in achalasia esophagus, a disorder in which LES relaxation is impaired and there is no peristalsis in the circular muscle.[34] In achalasia esophagus, swallow induces simultaneous pressure increase throughout the length of the esophagus, which is also termed as common cavity pressure or esophageal pressurization (**Fig. 5**). Concurrent HRM and US imaging reveal that pressurization of the esophagus is actually the results of another unique longitudinal muscle contraction pattern, in which longitudinal muscle contracts in the distal esophagus (similar to transient LES relaxation). Latter causes axial shortening of the esophagus and decrease in esophageal luminal cross-sectional area, both of which reduce esophageal volume. Because esophagus is closed at the 2 ends (by upper esophageal sphincter and LES), reduction in esophageal volume leads to a proportional increase in the pressure (Boyles law of physics), which manifests as common cavity or pressurization of the esophagus. It is clear that esophageal pressurization caused by longitudinal muscle contraction is a crucial factor in whatever little swallow-induced esophageal emptying occurs in patients with achalasia esophagus.

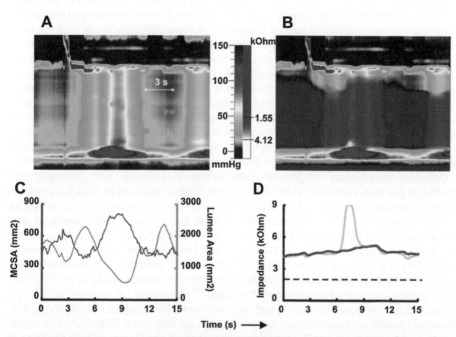

Fig. 5. Longitudinal muscle contraction in Type 2 achalasia esophagus. Simultaneous HRM, impedance, and US image–recorded changes in esophageal lumen and MCSA in a patient with type 2 achalasia: (*A*) HRM alone, (*B*) HRM and impedance, (*C*) changes in MCSA and lumen (derived from US images), and (*D*) impedance recording from a pair of electrodes above and below the esophagogastric junction (EGJ). Following swallow, there is a simultaneous pressure wave throughout the length of the esophagus (common cavity wave; panesophageal pressurization). EGJ record shows minimal relaxation to contraction following swallow. Impedance recording shows no flow across the EGJ. US image–derived data show a decrease in luminal CSA and increase in MCSA during the period of common cavity pressure wave (panesophageal pressurization). The increase in MCSA suggests contraction of the longitudinal muscle of the esophagus. (*From* Hong SJ, Bhargava V, Jiang Y, et al. A unique esophageal motor pattern that involves longitudinal muscles is responsible for emptying in achalasia esophagus. Gastroenterology 2010;139:102–11; with permission.)

Based on the swallow-induced esophageal pressure patterns seen with high-resolution manometry, achalasia has been divided into 3 types: Type 1 with minimal pressurization of esophagus, type 2 in which esophageal pressurization exceeds 30 mm Hg, and type 3 with a spastic type of esophageal contraction.[35] Several studies show that among different types of achalasia, type 2 respond best to treatment (botox injection, pneumatic dilation, or surgery).[35–37] It turns out that the longitudinal muscle contraction patterns are also quite different in 3 types of achalasia.[34] Type 1 achalasia shows minimal or no longitudinal muscle contraction; in type 2, strong longitudinal muscle contractions occur with swallows; and in type 3 there is severe discoordination between the 2 muscle layers. It may be that robust longitudinal muscle contraction in type 2 achalasia, which is largely responsible for esophageal pressurization and emptying, is a reason for the good response to medical/surgical therapy in type 2 achalasia in contrast to type 1 and type 3 achalasia patterns.

Eosinophilic esophagitis, a disease entity that is being diagnosed with increasing frequency since 1990s is caused by allergy to various food constituents.[38] Increase in numbers of eosinophils (>20 eosinophils/high-power field) in the esophageal mucosa is a hallmark histologic feature of eosinophilic esophagitis.[39] Dysphagia, the major symptom of eosinophilic esophagitis, is thought to result from narrowing of the esophagus due to eosinophil-induced submucosal fibrosis. Studies show that there is decrease in esophageal compliance in patients with eosinophilic esophagitis.[40] Esophageal manometry, which measures circular muscle contraction, is relatively normal in most patients with eosinophilic esophagitis. On the other hand, US imaging study shows that the longitudinal muscle function is severely impaired in these patients.[17] Latter manifests as reduced amplitude of longitudinal muscle contraction, discoordination between the 2 muscle layers, and reduced response to cholinergic agents. It is very possible that longitudinal muscle dysfunction leads to impaired descending relaxation, which manifests as relative narrowing on the radiologic studies and reduced esophageal wall compliance on the functional (functional luminal imaging probe [FLIP]) studies.

Cause of esophageal "anginalike" pain (pressure, squeeze, and tightness) and heartburn (burning sensation in the retrosternal region) resistant to acid suppression therapy remains elusive. In the era of over-the-counter proton pump inhibitors (PPIs), physicians, especial specialists, seldom see patients with heartburn and esophageal pain in their clinics that is responsive to PPI therapy. Prolonged manometry studies in the 1980s and early 1990s excluded esophageal spasm as the cause of "anginalike" pain. Current thinking is that "noncardiac" pain and PPI-resistant heartburn are related to hypersensitivity of the esophagus (hypersensitivity to acid, esophageal distension, and other physiologic stimuli).[41] Prolonged US imaging recordings reveal a close temporal correlation between sustained (prolonged) contraction of longitudinal muscle and esophageal pain[19] as well as heartburn (**Fig. 6**).[42] The mean duration of contraction was 70 seconds in the case of chest pain and 33 seconds in the case of heartburn in these studies. It may be that longitudinal muscle spasm is actually the cause of esophageal pain and PPI-resistant heartburn. Because prolonged US imaging studies are not practical (equipment is expensive and data analysis is cumbersome), alternative strategies are needed to demonstrate the cause and effect of relationship between longitudinal muscle spasm and esophageal pain. One such possibility is prolonged ambulatory high-resolution manometry that can detect cranial lift of the LES as a marker of longitudinal muscle contraction. The feasibility of this approach has recently been demonstrated.[43] How does prolonged contraction of the longitudinal muscle cause esophageal pain/heartburn is not known but it clearly reduces esophageal wall blood perfusion as discussed in the section of laser Doppler flow monitoring of the esophageal wall.

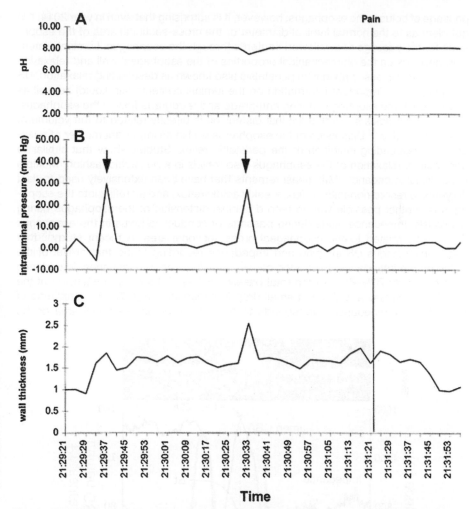

Fig. 6. Sustained esophageal contraction associated with chest pain. Esophageal pH (*A*), distal esophageal pressure (*B*), and esophageal smooth muscle thickness (*C*) are shown during a 2.5-minute recorded interval. The onset of chest pain is depicted by the vertical line (time = 0). The onset of sustained esophageal contraction (SEC) occurs approximately 120 seconds before the onset of pain. The pressure record shows 2 small contractions (*arrows*) that are accompanied by brief increases in esophageal muscle thickness during the SEC. (*From* Balaban DH, Yamamoto Y, Liu J, et al. Sustained esophageal contraction: a marker of esophageal chest pain identified by intraluminal ultrasonography. Gastroenterology 1999;116:29–37; with permission.)

LUMINAL DISTENSION MEASUREMENT BY US IMAGING AND IMPEDANCE RECORDINGS

Distension of esophagus during passage of bolus is an important parameter that is somewhat difficult to measure. It is important because the flow through a tube is directly related to its cross-sectional area and therefore it is not difficult to imagine that if the esophagus did not distend well it would lead to difficulty swallowing or dysphagia. Barium swallow study provides information on the luminal diameter during passage of bolus in the esophagus; however, it is surprising that even in year 2014, it is not clear as to the normal luminal diameter or the cross-sectional area of the esophagus for the passage of swallowed contents through the esophagus. Luminal distension depends on the biomechanical properties of the esophageal wall and relaxation of the muscle in association with peristalsis also known as descending relaxation. US images provide important information on the luminal contents (air, liquid) as well as distension of the esophagus during antegrade and retrograde flow in the esophagus. US imaging studies show that luminal distension is directly related to the volume of swallowed bolus.[44] Distension of the esophagus is also an important marker of relaxation or descending inhibition of the peristaltic reflex. Studies show that similar to contraction, relaxation of the esophagus also travels in a peristaltic fashion. Multiple intraluminal impedance (MII) measurements that have been extensively used for last 20 years to record nonacidic reflux, weakly acidic reflux, and air reflux into the esophagus is another possible way to record luminal distension of the esophagus during peristalsis. Impedance value during passage of conductive bolus in the esophagus is inversely related to the esophageal cross-sectional area. A recent study[45] that used simultaneous US imaging and impedance recording found that arrival of the bolus on the impedance electrodes causes a major drop in esophageal impedance (approximately 70%–80% of the total baseline value). Subsequent distension of the esophagus causes a further but small drop in impedance (**Fig. 7**). The amplitude of small drop in impedance corresponds to the luminal cross- sectional area or the

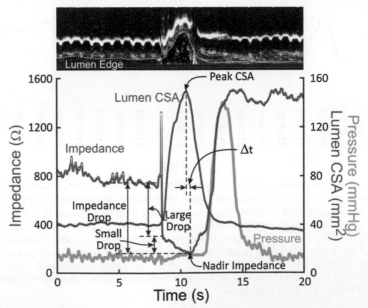

Fig. 7. Temporal correlation between changes in luminal CSA and changes in impedance values. A B-mode US image is shown on the top of the graph and it shows changes in luminal CSA over time on one side of the US probe. An increase in impedance coincides with the passage of air through the esophagus, followed by a large drop in impedance with the onset of increase in luminal CSA, which was followed by a slow decrease in impedance associated with the increase in the luminal CSA. Peak cross-sectional area coincides approximately with the nadir impedance. (*From* Kim JH, Mittal RK, Patel N, et al. Esophageal distension during bolus transport: can it be detected by intraluminal impedance recordings? Neurogastroenterol Motil 2014;26:1122–30; with permission.)

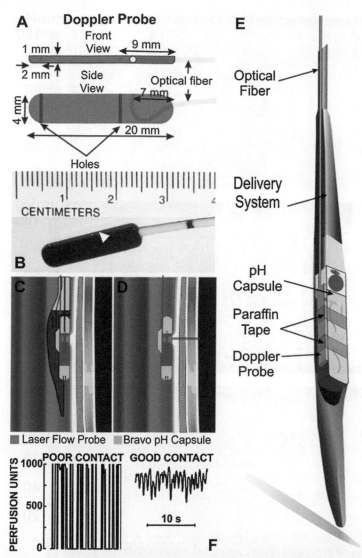

Fig. 8. Laser Doppler technique to record blood perfusion of the esophageal wall. (*A*) Laser Doppler probe; (*B*) the Doppler probe with scale in background; (*C, D*) Bravo and laser Doppler probe anchored to the esophageal wall—Laser Doppler probe was taped to the Bravo pH capsule. Using the Bravo pH delivery system (*C*) the capsule was anchored to the esophageal wall and delivery system was removed (*D*). (*E*) Laser Doppler perfusion recordings when capsule was inadequately fixed to the esophageal wall (poor contact) and (*F*) when properly anchored. With poor contact the recordings yield artifact but with good contact a stable recording can be obtained continuously for hours. (*From* Jiang Y, Bhargava V, Kim YS, et al. Esophageal wall blood perfusion during contraction and transient lower esophageal sphincter relaxation in humans. Am J Physiol Gastrointest Liver Physiol 2012;303:G529–35; with permission.)

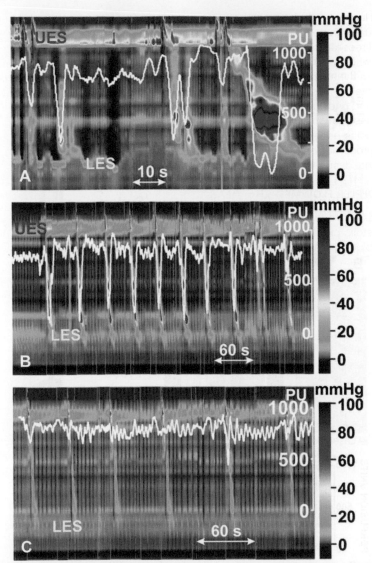

Fig. 9. Esophageal wall perfusion during swallow induced esophageal contractions: Doppler perfusion tracings are superimposed white line on the high-resolution manometry tracings. Doppler transducer was taped to the Bravo pH capsule, which was anchored 4 to 6 cm above the lower esophageal sphincter. (*A*) The decrease in laser Doppler perfusion with each swallow induced esophageal contraction. Amplitude and duration of perfusion record is related to the amplitude and duration of esophageal contraction. (*B*) The effect of wet swallow-induced esophageal wall contraction on the reduction in esophageal wall perfusion. (*C*) The effect of atropine on the laser Doppler perfusion during wet swallow. Atropine reduced the esophageal contraction amplitude and reduction in blood perfusion with esophageal contractions. (*From* Jiang Y, Bhargava V, Kim YS, et al. Esophageal wall blood perfusion during contraction and transient lower esophageal sphincter relaxation in humans. Am J Physiol Gastrointest Liver Physiol 2012;303:G529–35; with permission.)

degree of luminal distension. Following swallow of a conductive solution, nadir imped-ance occurs with peak luminal distension. MII recordings show that nadir impedance on the MII recordings travel in a peristaltic fashion, from oral to aboral end during peri-stalsis,[46] which confirms that with swallow-induced peristalsis, similar to contraction, inhibition of the esophagus also travels in a peristaltic fashion. One can also measure luminal distension associated with reflux (GER) during transient LES relaxation with US imaging, and one such study found that some of chest pain episodes related to GER occur in association with large volume reflex and marked esophageal distension.[47] Future studies need to assess if poor luminal distension, whether related to biome-chanical properties of the esophageal wall or poor descending relaxation is the cause of functional dysphagia, also referred to as nonobstructive dysphagia.

LASER DOPPLER FLOWMETRY TO MEASURE ESOPHAGEAL WALL BLOOD PERFUSION

The blood flows into the myocardium during diastolic phase of cardiac cycle because during systolic phase myocardial contraction constricts/occludes blood vessels and prevents blood from entering into the myocardium. A similar phenomenon was found in the stomach.[48] Along the same lines, recent studies show that during swallow-induced esophageal contractions (primary peristalsis) there is almost complete cessa-tion of the esophageal wall perfusion (**Figs. 8** and **9**).[49,50] Remember, during peristalsis circular and longitudinal muscles contract simultaneously. Transient LES relaxation that is associated with esophageal longitudinal muscle contraction is also associated with significant reduction in the esophageal wall perfusion. These observations raise possibility that prolonged contractions of longitudinal muscles of the esophagus (sus-tained esophageal wall contraction) could lead to ischemia of esophageal wall and, similar to myocardial pain, "anginalike" esophageal pain may result from esophageal wall ischemia. Laser Doppler recording require that the laser Doppler probe is anchored to the esophageal wall so that the laser beam stay directed toward the esophageal wall. We used Bravo probe delivery system to anchor the laser Doppler probe to the esophageal wall and using such a system they recorded esophageal wall perfusion for extended time periods (see **Fig. 9**). Interestingly, the recordings appear similar to pH recordings and therefore are amenable to relatively easy data analysis. Future studies will be able to answer question whether esophageal wall ischemia is an important cause of esophageal pain and PPI-resistant heartburn/chest pain.

SUMMARY

Esophagus is a simple organ, a relative straight tube with relatively simple function, that is, to transfer the swallowed contents into the stomach or in the other opposite direction during reflux, belching, and vomiting. Diversity of the techniques available to test esophageal function described in this issue of "Clinics of North America" is a testament that may be it is not that simple of an organ and may be our understanding of its functioning is not yet complete. Cause of dysphagia remains obscure in large number of patients. Dysphagia in the setting of normal endoscopy, barium swallow study, and manometry is labeled as functional dysphagia. From a mechanical point of view, for transfer of material through a tube only 2 things are important: the diameter/cross-sectional area of a tube and driving pressure or pressure gradients along the length of the tube. HRM is almost a perfect tool to measure driving pressures and pressure gradients across the tube. On the other hand, the author believes none of the available technique provides accurate measurement of the cross-sectional area of the esophagus during bolus transport. FLIP can measure the relationship between esophageal pressure and cross-sectional of the esophagus during induced distension of the esophagus but not during bolus transport. Dynamic US imaging of the esophagus can measure luminal dimensions during bolus transport but there are limitations, that is, equipment is expensive, swallowed air causes disruption of esophageal imaging, image analysis is time consuming, and one can only obtain information at one level in the esophagus at a given time unless one uses multiple US probes. Barium swallow or esophagram provides approximation of esophageal diameter during bolus transport but there are limitations. MII has been mostly used to detect weakly acidic and nonacidic reflux but work of Omari and colleagues[41,46] show that MII can detect luminal dimension during bolus transport. Our recent study shows that there is an inverse but statistically significant linear relationship between the esophageal cross-sectional area and impedance value. If MII technique can be further developed along these lines, it could add significantly to our diagnostic armamentarium because HRM Z (manometry + impedance) is easy to record and number of recording systems are already available.

"Anginalike" esophageal pain and heartburn nonresponsive to PPI therapy are major health care issues and consume tremendous amount of health care resources. The precise pathogenesis of these symptoms is highly debated. We have excellent methodologies to diagnose acid and nonacid reflux but it is clear that reflux is not the cause of the symptoms in most of these patients. Current thinking is that "esophageal hypersensitivity" is the cause of these symptoms, which implies that normal stimuli, such as low levels of esophageal distension, normal amount of acid reflux, and even normal esophageal contractions, are felt as pain by these patients. One possibility is that the commonly used esophageal function testing does not record the actual culprit or the offending stimulus. May be it is the longitudinal muscle spasm that is the cause of esophageal pain but and as pointed out earlier it is not easy to record. Because esophageal pain and heartburn occurs intermittently and infrequently, one requires prolonged, ambulatory monitoring technique, such as ambulatory HRM to detect LES lift/esophageal shortening as a marker of longitudinal muscle spasm. Our recent work indicates that longitudinal muscle contraction can cause low esophageal wall blood perfusion. If future studies prove that ischemia of the esophageal wall is an important cause of esophageal pain, laser Doppler flowmetry could become an important tool in the esophageal function testing laboratories across the country very quickly.

REFERENCES

1. Gilbert RJ, Gaige TA, Wang R, et al. Resolving the three-dimensional myoarchitecture of bovine esophageal wall with diffusion spectrum imaging and tractography. Cell Tissue Res 2008;332:461–8.
2. Dai Q, Korimilli A, Thangada VK, et al. Muscle shortening along the normal esophagus during swallowing. Dig Dis Sci 2006;51:105–9.
3. Vegesna AK, Chuang KY, Besetty R, et al. Circular smooth muscle contributes to esophageal shortening during peristalsis. World J Gastroenterol 2012;18:4317–22.
4. Nicosia MA, Brasseur JG, Liu JB, et al. Local longitudinal muscle shortening of the human esophagus from high-frequency ultrasonography. Am J Physiol Gastrointest Liver Physiol 2001;281:G1022–33.
5. Sugarbaker DJ, Rattan S, Goyal RK. Swallowing induces sequential activation of esophageal longitudinal smooth muscle. Am J Physiol 1984;247:G515–9.
6. Pouderoux P, Lin S, Kahrilas PJ. Timing, propagation, coordination, and effect of esophageal shortening during peristalsis. Gastroenterology 1997;112:1147–54.

7. Edmundowicz SA, Clouse RE. Shortening of the esophagus in response to swallowing. Am J Physiol 1991;260:G512–6.
8. Dodds WJ, Stewart ET, Hodges D, et al. Movement of the feline esophagus associated with respiration and peristalsis. An evaluation using tantalum markers. J Clin Invest 1973;52:1–13.
9. Lee Y, Whiting J, Robertson E, et al. Measuring movement and location of the gastroesophageal junction:research and clinical implications. Scand J Gastroenterol 2013;48:401–11.
10. Miller LS, Liu JB, Colizzo FP, et al. Correlation of high-frequency esophageal ultrasonography and manometry in the study of esophageal motility. Gastroenterology 1995;109:832–7.
11. Mittal RK, Liu J, Puckett JL, et al. Sensory and motor function of the esophagus: lessons from ultrasound imaging. Gastroenterology 2005;128:487–97.
12. Puckett JL, Bhalla V, Liu J, et al. Oesophageal wall stress and muscle hypertrophy in high amplitude oesophageal contractions. Neurogastroenterol Motil 2005;17: 791–9.
13. Mittal RK, Kassab G, Puckett JL, et al. Hypertrophy of the muscularis propria of the lower esophageal sphincter and the body of the esophagus in patients with primary motility disorders of the esophagus. Am J Gastroenterol 2003;98:1705–12.
14. Takeda T, Kassab G, Liu J, et al. Effect of atropine on the biomechanical properties of the oesophageal wall in humans. J Physiol 2003;547:621–8.
15. Dogan I, Puckett JL, Padda BS, et al. Prevalence of increased esophageal muscle thickness in patients with esophageal symptoms. Am J Gastroenterol 2007; 102:137–45.
16. Li C, Kuemmerle JF. Mechanisms that mediate the development of fibrosis in patients with Crohn's disease. Inflamm Bowel Dis 2014;20:1250–8.
17. Korsapati H, Babaei A, Bhargava V, et al. Dysfunction of the longitudinal muscles of the oesophagus in eosinophilic oesophagitis. Gut 2009;58:1056–62.
18. Miller LS, Liu JB, Klenn PJ, et al. Endoluminal ultrasonography of the distal esophagus in systemic sclerosis. Gastroenterology 1993;105:31–9.
19. Balaban DH, Yamamoto Y, Liu J, et al. Sustained esophageal contraction: a marker of esophageal chest pain identified by intraluminal ultrasonography. Gastroenterology 1999;116:29–37.
20. Mittal RK, Padda B, Bhalla V, et al. Synchrony between circular and longitudinal muscle contractions during peristalsis in normal subjects. Am J Physiol Gastrointest Liver Physiol 2006;290:G431–8.
21. Clouse RE, Staiano A. Topography of normal and high-amplitude esophageal peristalsis. Am J Physiol 1993;265:G1098–107.
22. Yamamoto Y, Liu J, Smith TK, et al. Distension-related responses in circular and longitudinal muscle of the human esophagus: an ultrasonographic study. Am J Physiol 1998;275:G805–11.
23. Babaei A, Bhargava V, Korsapati H, et al. A unique longitudinal muscle contraction pattern associated with transient lower esophageal sphincter relaxation. Gastroenterology 2008;134:1322–31.
24. Pandolfino JE, Zhang QG, Ghosh SK, et al. Transient lower esophageal sphincter relaxations and reflux: mechanistic analysis using concurrent fluoroscopy and high-resolution manometry. Gastroenterology 2006;131:1725–33.
25. Leslie E, Bhargava V, Mittal RK. A novel pattern of longitudinal muscle contraction with subthreshold pharyngeal stimulus: a possible mechanism of lower esophageal sphincter relaxation. Am J Physiol Gastrointest Liver Physiol 2012; 302:G542–7.

26. Pal A, Brasseur JG. The mechanical advantage of local longitudinal shortening on peristaltic transport. J Biomech Eng 2002;124:94–100.
27. Dogan I, Bhargava V, Liu J, et al. Axial stretch: a novel mechanism of the lower esophageal sphincter relaxation. Am J Physiol Gastrointest Liver Physiol 2007; 292:G329–34.
28. Jiang Y, Bhargava V, Mittal RK. Mechanism of stretch-activated excitatory and inhibitory responses in the lower esophageal sphincter. Am J Physiol Gastrointest Liver Physiol 2009;297:G397–405.
29. Abrahao L Jr, Bhargava V, Babaei A, et al. Swallow induces a peristaltic wave of distension that marches in front of the peristaltic wave of contraction. Neurogastroenterol Motil 2011;23:201–7, e110.
30. Korsapati H, Babaei A, Bhargava V, et al. Cholinergic stimulation induces asynchrony between the circular and longitudinal muscle contraction during esophageal peristalsis. Am J Physiol Gastrointest Liver Physiol 2008;294:G694–8.
31. Jung HY, Puckett JL, Bhalla V, et al. Asynchrony between the circular and the longitudinal muscle contraction in patients with nutcracker esophagus. Gastroenterology 2005;128:1179–86.
32. Korsapati H, Bhargava V, Mittal RK. Reversal of asynchrony between circular and longitudinal muscle contraction in nutcracker esophagus by atropine. Gastroenterology 2008;135:796–802.
33. Kim HS, Park H, Lim JH, et al. Morphometric evaluation of oesophageal wall in patients with nutcracker oesophagus and ineffective oesophageal motility. Neurogastroenterol Motil 2008;20:869–76.
34. Hong SJ, Bhargava V, Jiang Y, et al. A unique esophageal motor pattern that involves longitudinal muscles is responsible for emptying in achalasia esophagus. Gastroenterology 2010;139:102–11.
35. Pandolfino JE, Kwiatek MA, Nealis T, et al. Achalasia: a new clinically relevant classification by high-resolution manometry. Gastroenterology 2008;135:1526–33.
36. Rohof WO, Hirsch DP, Kessing BF, et al. Efficacy of treatment for patients with achalasia depends on the distensibility of the esophagogastric junction. Gastroenterology 2012;143:328–35.
37. Rohof WO, Salvador R, Annese V, et al. Outcomes of treatment for achalasia depend on manometric subtype. Gastroenterology 2013;144:718–25.
38. Gonsalves N, Yang GY, Doerfler B, et al. Elimination diet effectively treats eosinophilic esophagitis in adults; food reintroduction identifies causative factors. Gastroenterology 2012;142:1451–9.e1 [quiz: e14–5].
39. Furuta GT, Liacouras CA, Collins MH, et al. Eosinophilic esophagitis in children and adults: a systematic review and consensus recommendations for diagnosis and treatment. Gastroenterology 2007;133:1342–63.
40. Kwiatek MA, Hirano I, Kahrilas PJ, et al. Mechanical properties of the esophagus in eosinophilic esophagitis. Gastroenterology 2011;140:82–90.
41. Miwa H, Kondo T, Oshima T, et al. Esophageal sensation and esophageal hypersensitivity - overview from bench to bedside. J Neurogastroenterol Motil 2010; 16:353–62.
42. Pehlivanov N, Liu J, Mittal RK. Sustained esophageal contraction: a motor correlate of heartburn symptom. Am J Physiol Gastrointest Liver Physiol 2001;281: G743–51.
43. Mittal RK, Karstens A, Leslie E, et al. Ambulatory high-resolution manometry, lower esophageal sphincter lift and transient lower esophageal sphincter relaxation. Neurogastroenterol Motil 2012;24:40–6, e2.

44. Rhee PL, Liu J, Puckett JL, et al. Measuring esophageal distension by high-frequency intraluminal ultrasound probe. Am J Physiol Gastrointest Liver Physiol 2002;283:G886–92.
45. Kim HJ, Mittal RK, Patel N, et al. Esophageal distension during bolus transport: can it be detected by intraluminal impedance recordings? Neurogastroenterol Motil 2014;26(8):1122–30.
46. Nguyen NQ, Holloway RH, Smout AJ, et al. Automated impedance-manometry analysis detects esophageal motor dysfunction in patients who have non-obstructive dysphagia with normal manometry. Neurogastroenterol Motil 2013; 25:238–45, e164.
47. Tipnis NA, Rhee PL, Mittal RK. Distension during gastroesophageal reflux: effects of acid inhibition and correlation with symptoms. Am J Physiol Gastrointest Liver Physiol 2007;293:G469–74.
48. Livingston EH, Howard TJ, Garrick TR, et al. Strong gastric contractions cause mucosal ischemia. Am J Physiol 1991;260:G524–30.
49. Jiang Y, Bhargava V, Kim YS, et al. Esophageal wall blood perfusion during contraction and transient lower esophageal sphincter relaxation in humans. Am J Physiol Gastrointest Liver Physiol 2012;303:G529–35.
50. Mittal RK, Bhargava V, Lal H, et al. Effect of esophageal contraction on esophageal wall blood perfusion. Am J Physiol Gastrointest Liver Physiol 2011;301: G1093–8.

Index

Note: Page numbers of article titles are in **boldface** type.

A

Achalasia, 612–614, 644–645
  barium esophagography in, 572–574
  impedance planimetry in, 613–614
  treatment of, persistent dysphagia after, 645–646
  types of, 676
Achalasia esophagus, muscle contraction in, 675
Antireflex surgery, dysphagia following, 650
Aperistalsis, 554

B

Baristat balloon testing, provocative, in gastrointestinal tract, 623–625
Barium esophagography, advantages of, 564–566
  esoophagram in, 564
  introduction of, 563
  performance of, 564
  role of, in endoscopy world, **563–580**
  terminology used in, 563–564
  to describe esophageal physiology, 579
  use in specific esophageal disorders, 566–574
  video swallow study in, 564
Barium radiography, compared with endoscopy, theoretic advantages of, 564–566
  principles of, 564
Belching, 633
Belching disorders, and rumination syndrome, esophageal function testing for, **633–642**
  clinical evaluation and diagnosis of, 637–639
  pathophysiology of, 637
  treatment of, 639–640
Bolus transit, esophageal, impedance monitoring of, **595–605**
    validation of, 596–598
Brain imaging, to assess esophageal sensation, 627–628

C

Caustic injury of esophagus, barium esophagography in, 575–576
Chest pain, noncardiac, provocative testing in, 623
Chicago Classification, abnormalies of esophageal peristalsis defined by, 556–557
  as evolving process, 558
  dysphagia associated with motility disorders defined in, 644–649
  limitations of, 557
  of motility disorders, **545–561**
  swallow pattern and metrics characterization, 546

Gastrointest Endoscopy Clin N Am 24 (2014) 687–692
http://dx.doi.org/10.1016/S1052-5157(14)00083-X
1052-5157/14/$ – see front matter © 2014 Elsevier Inc. All rights reserved.

United States Postal Service

Statement of Ownership, Management, and Circulation
(All Periodicals Publications Except Requester Publications)

1. Publication Title	2. Publication Number	3. Filing Date
Gastrointestinal Endoscopy Clinics of North America	0 1 2 - 6 0 3	9/14/14

4. Issue Frequency	5. Number of Issues Published Annually	6. Annual Subscription Price
Jan, Apr, Jul, Oct	4	$335.00

7. Complete Mailing Address of Known Office of Publication (Not printer) (Street, city, county, state, and ZIP+4®)

Elsevier Inc.
360 Park Avenue South
New York, NY 10010-1710

Contact Person
Stephen R. Bushing

Telephone (Include area code)
215-239-3688

8. Complete Mailing Address of Headquarters or General Business Office of Publisher (Not printer)

Elsevier Inc., 360 Park Avenue South, New York, NY 10010-1710

9. Full Names and Complete Mailing Addresses of Publisher, Editor, and Managing Editor (Do not leave blank)

Publisher (Name and complete mailing address)

Linda Belfus, Elsevier Inc., 1600 John F. Kennedy Blvd., Suite 1800, Philadelphia, PA 19103-2899

Editor (Name and complete mailing address)

Kerry Holland, Elsevier Inc., 1600 John F. Kennedy Blvd., Suite 1800, Philadelphia, PA 19103-2899

Managing Editor (Name and complete mailing address)

Adrianne Brigido, Elsevier Inc., 1600 John F. Kennedy Blvd., Suite 1800, Philadelphia, PA 19103-2899

10. Owner (Do not leave blank. If the publication is owned by a corporation, give the name and address of the corporation immediately followed by the names and addresses of all stockholders owning or holding 1 percent or more of the total amount of stock. If not owned by a corporation, give the names and addresses of the individual owners. If owned by a partnership or other unincorporated firm, give its name and address as well as those of each individual owner. If the publication is published by a nonprofit organization, give its name and address.)

Full Name	Complete Mailing Address
Wholly owned subsidiary of	1600 John F. Kennedy Blvd. Ste. 1800
Reed/Elsevier, US holdings	Philadelphia, PA 19103-2899

11. Known Bondholders, Mortgagees, and Other Security Holders Owning or Holding 1 Percent or More of Total Amount of Bonds, Mortgages, or Other Securities. If none, check box ☐ None

Full Name	Complete Mailing Address
N/A	

12. Tax Status (For completion by nonprofit organizations authorized to mail at nonprofit rates) (Check one)
The purpose, function, and nonprofit status of this organization and the exempt status for federal income tax purposes:
☐ Has Not Changed During Preceding 12 Months
☐ Has Changed During Preceding 12 Months (Publisher must submit explanation of change with this statement)

PS Form 3526, August 2012 (Page 1 of 3 (Instructions Page 3)) PSN 7530-01-000-9931 PRIVACY NOTICE: See our Privacy policy in www.usps.com

---

13. Publication Title	14. Issue Date for Circulation Data Below
Gastrointestinal Endoscopy Clinics of North America	July 2014

15. Extent and Nature of Circulation			Average No. Copies Each Issue During Preceding 12 Months	No. Copies of Single Issue Published Nearest to Filing Date
a. Total Number of Copies (Net press run)			454	489
b. Paid Circulation (By Mail and Outside the Mail)	(1)	Mailed Outside-County Paid Subscriptions Stated on PS Form 3541. (Include paid distribution above nominal rate, advertiser's proof copies, and exchange copies)	227	235
	(2)	Mailed In-County Paid Subscriptions Stated on PS Form 3541 (Include paid distribution above nominal rate, advertiser's proof copies, and exchange copies)		
	(3)	Paid Distribution Outside the Mails Including Sales Through Dealers and Carriers, Street Vendors, Counter Sales, and Other Paid Distribution Outside USPS®	66	70
	(4)	Paid Distribution by Other Classes Mailed Through the USPS (e.g. First-Class Mail®)		
c. Total Paid Distribution (Sum of 15b (1), (2), (3), and (4))		▲	293	305
d. Free or Nominal Rate Distribution (By Mail and Outside the Mail)	(1)	Free or Nominal Rate Outside-County Copies Included on PS Form 3541	61	84
	(2)	Free or Nominal Rate In-County Copies Included on PS Form 3541		
	(3)	Free or Nominal Rate Copies Mailed at Other Classes Through the USPS (e.g. First-Class Mail)		
	(4)	Free or Nominal Rate Distribution Outside the Mail (Carriers or other means)		
e. Total Free or Nominal Rate Distribution (Sum of 15d (1), (2), (3) and (4))		▲	61	84
f. Total Distribution (Sum of 15c and 15e)		▲	354	389
g. Copies not Distributed (See instructions to publishers #4 (page #3))		▲	100	100
h. Total (Sum of 15f and g)		▲	454	489
i. Percent Paid (15c divided by 15f times 100)		▲	82.77%	78.41%

16. Total circulation includes electronic copies. Report circulation on PS Form 3526-X worksheet.

17. Publication of Statement of Ownership
If the publication is a general publication, publication of this statement is required. Will be printed in the October 2014 issue of this publication.

18. Signature and Title of Editor, Publisher, Business Manager, or Owner

Stephen R. Bushing – Inventory Distribution Coordinator

Date
September 14, 2014

I certify that all information furnished on this form is true and complete. I understand that anyone who furnishes false or misleading information on this form or who omits material or information requested on the form may be subject to criminal sanctions (including fines and imprisonment) and/or civil sanctions (including civil penalties).

PS Form 3526, August 2012 (Page 2 of 3)

Moving?

Make sure your subscription moves with you!

To notify us of your new address, find your **Clinics Account Number** (located on your mailing label above your name), and contact customer service at:

Email: journalscustomerservice-usa@elsevier.com

800-654-2452 (subscribers in the U.S. & Canada)
314-447-8871 (subscribers outside of the U.S. & Canada)

Fax number: 314-447-8029

Elsevier Health Sciences Division
Subscription Customer Service
3251 Riverport Lane
Maryland Heights, MO 63043

*To ensure uninterrupted delivery of your subscription, please notify us at least 4 weeks in advance of move.

ELSEVIER

Printed and bound by CPI Group (UK) Ltd, Croydon, CR0 4YY

03/10/2024

01040490-0016